Dr. Jo's

# No
# Big
# Deal
# Diet

*seven skills for successful weight loss*

# Joanne V. Lichten, PhD, RD

# Nutrifit Publishing

# Dr. Jo's No Big Deal Diet

## Joanne V. Lichten, PhD, RD

**Published by:**
Nutrifit Publishing
PO Box 669144
Marietta, GA  30066
770-973-6242
Email: contact@drjo.com
www.drjo.com

Printed in the USA
Cover design by Elizabeth Piarote

Publisher's Cataloging-in-Publication

Lichten, Joanne V.
   Dr. Jo's No Big Deal Diet/Joanne V. Lichten
(aka Dr. Jo).
--1st ed.
p. cm.
No Big Deal Diet
Cover title: Dr. Jo's No Big Deal Diet
ISBN: 1-880347-45-8

1. Diet.   I. Title.   II. Title: No Big Deal Diet.   III. Title: Dr Jo's No Big Deal Diet.   IV. Author: Dr Jo

***Have you ever said:***

- ☐ "I just can't seem to lose weight."
- ☐ "I've lost weight lots of times - I just can't keep it off."
- ☐ "Sometimes my eating is out-of-control."
- ☐ "I'm tired of dieting - eating the same foods and always feeling deprived."
- ☐ "I'll never lose weight - I just don't have the *willpower* to stick to a program."
- ☐ "I know more about diet and exercise than my body demonstrates."

If you checked off even one of the above statements, *Dr. Jo's No Big Deal Diet* can help you! As a registered dietitian for more than 25 years, I have helped thousands of patients get their weight under control. In my research with people who had lost weight and kept it off - I've discovered three truths about successful weight loss:

1. Knowledge alone does not make healthy changes. If you checked off the last statement, *Dr. Jo's No Big Deal Diet* will help you bridge from *knowing* it to actually *doing* it!

2. There is no *one* perfect diet. But there is at least one way to lose weight that is perfect for *you*! And, I'll help you discover it for yourself.

3. You don't need *will*power to successfully lose weight and keep it off. People who have been successful at losing weight and keeping it off didn't have any more willpower than others. Instead, they used *skill*power by practicing seven specific skills that kept their weight in control.

It really *is* "No Big Deal" to lose weight, get your eating under control, and keep the excess weight off forever. *Dr. Jo's No Big Deal Diet* is about discovering and practicing the seven skills that will help you. I have faith, that you too, will be successful!

Dr Jo

# Table of Contents

Introduction:

# Getting Started

Have you heard the statistic that 95% of all diets fail? For every 100 people who go on a diet, 95 will gain back all the weight they had lost. Depressing, isn't it? No wonder many of us say, "Why even bother? I'll just gain it back!"

This oft-quoted statistic combined with our personal experience of repeated, unsuccessful attempts to lose weight can be very disheartening. After so many failures, some people just stop trying. The chronic dieter, on the other hand, will keep looking for their next magic program, potion, or pill. They begin the cycle of trying and failing, and trying and failing. No wonder many of us have low self-esteem when it comes to our bodies. To cheer you up, let me share with you, as Paul Harvey calls it, "The Rest of the Story."

# Dr. Jo's No Big Deal Diet

## The Optimistic News about Successful Weight Loss

The statistic that 95% of all diets fail doesn't tell us the whole story. First, this research comes from University-run weight loss programs with hard-core dieters. The University-run programs often have structured programs not much different than the ones we see advertised on television and in the newspaper.

But guess what? The majority of *successful* dieters do not lose weight using organized weight loss programs. Many studies, including my own, have revealed that most people that are successful with weight loss have lost it on their own. They may have used information that they learned from previous attempts, but their last successful weight loss attempt is often self-initiated and self-monitored. Let me quote a few studies:

- The Minnesota Heart Survey (1984) found that while most people presently or formerly overweight had attempted dieting to lose weight, only 47% enrolled in a formal education program.
- Schachter (1982) found that more individuals lost their excess weight and maintained on their own rather than with a weight management program; only 30% sought professional assistance.
- Colvin and Olson (1983) interviewed only the successful dieters and found that 53% of males and 34% of the females followed a structured program for weight-loss.
- Lichten (1989) found that 81% of the Mexican American women who had lost weight had succeeded on their own.
- Fletcher (1994) interviewed 160 "masters" (those that had lost 20 pounds or more and kept it off for at least three years). More than half of these people lost the weight on their own.
- National Weight Control Registry (http://www.nwcr.ws/) is an ongoing project of Dr. James Hill of the University of Colorado and Dr. Rena Wing of the University of Pittsburgh. Since 1993 they have collected a database of nearly 5000 people who have been successful at maintaining a weight loss of at least 30

pounds for one year or longer. They have found that about 50% of participants lost weight on their own without any type of formal program or help.

A second reason why the 95% failure rate for dieters is misleading is that it is based on a single attempt. In other words, if 100 dieters enter a particular program, only five people (5%) will lose weight and keep it off. But statistics about weight loss should not be quoted according to just one attempt. Who can do anything successfully from just one attempt? Do babies learn to walk in a single attempt? How many times did you have to struggle with a new computer software program before it really sunk in? All athletes and Olympic gold-medal winners have many losses before their grand win.

It's no different with weight loss. It may take several (or many) attempts to lose weight, but if you continue to learn from each experience, you will eventually be successful at weight loss. In the long run, many people are successful at losing weight and keeping it off. Famous examples include weight-loss gurus Richard Simmons and Jane Brody (Personal Health Columnist, New York Times). You, too, can lose weight and keep it off if you learn from those who have been successful!

**Dr. Jo's Personal Struggle**

The reason I wrote this book about successful weight loss is because I, too, struggled with my weight for many years. I had an eating disorder for five years and then spent many more years getting it under control. When I was just 16, I weighed about what I do now. I would now say that I was at an average weight for a female adult. But as a teenager, I felt chunky! I was always jealous of those girls who were barely five feet tall, very skinny, and very popular. I thought that if I were as thin as they were, my life would suddenly become more perfect.

# Dr. Jo's No Big Deal Diet

When I made the decision to do something about my "fat," I picked up some dieting tips in a young woman's magazine and initiated my first diet. It was actually a starvation diet. My diet for over almost a year consisted of half a grapefruit (without sugar, of course) for breakfast and a cup of hot water with a chicken bouillon for lunch.

After school I would have a cup of hot black tea and a piece of dry toast. Since dinner was always with my entire family, I ate what they did. But I took extremely small portions and ate very slowly (counting the number of chews) hoping that no one would notice – and because I was one of nine children they often didn't. After dinner, I would walk/run for at least an hour with my dog or do over an hour of laps in the swimming pool. Late in the evening I would escape to my bedroom where I would do a long routine of exercises including plenty of sit-ups and leg lifts for my "fat" belly!

Within a few months, I lost 40 pounds. At five feet six (and with a large bone structure including size ten shoes), I weighed under 100 pounds and thought I was beautiful. But unlike my hopes and dreams, I did not become more popular. In fact, I grew more shy and introverted. Probably because I was spending every waking moment thinking about how I would burn off that 60 calorie apple, how I could eat less at dinner, or escape someone's birthday cake without anyone noticing.

That 40 pound weight loss along with other physical symptoms and my extreme preoccupation with food would classify me as anorexic. But when my mother's concerns about my health sent me to the doctor, I denied that I had lost any weight at all. I kept the weight loss off my entire senior year but did not lose further. Because of the weight loss, I developed a severe intolerance to cold from which I still suffer.

The following year, I went away to college. As a freshman, I was required to live in the dormitory and use the all-you-can-eat cafeteria pass. And eat I did. In the beginning, I told myself that I was thin and deserved to have the desserts that I had not had for over a year. Unfortunately, I lost control at nearly every meal and ate until I was sick to my stomach. Then I hated myself for my lack of self-discipline. By the time I made my first trip back home from college, I had gained back nearly 30 pounds. My parents were pleased but I was not. I not only felt fat, but completely out of control. I knew I had to do something drastic.

That's when I began to experiment with every diet I read about, laxatives, self-induced vomiting, and periodic fasts. Every day for the next four years throughout college, I was either on a diet or losing control. When I got really disgusted at myself for losing control, I would fast for two or three days. Then I would convince myself that my eating was in control, my stomach had shrunk and now everything would be normal.

But it wasn't. Every moment of every day, I was thinking about what I wanted to eat, feeling guilty about what I had already eaten, or planning when I was going to start my next diet and how I would approach it. One of the diets I followed was the liquid protein diet. In fact, I was drinking my liquid protein one day when I heard on the radio: "16 people have died from the liquid protein diet." I remember looking at the very expensive protein supplement and internally debating as to whether I should take a chance and continue with the diet or throw it away. I finally poured it down the toilet, afraid that if I had put it in the trash I would later feel desperate and pull it back out.

Several times a week I would binge on 2000-3000+ calories of sweets at a time. Sometimes it was a whole box of what I had convinced myself was *healthy* granola. Othertimes it was a secret and elaborate ritual involving specific foods that were available between the dorm and the shopping mall.

Every weekend my friends and I would take the school bus to the mall. There, I'd eat a large, soft pretzel and an ice cream cone. While my friends would take the bus back to campus, I would elect to take the two-mile walk by myself. And on that walk, I would continue with my private fast food binge. I would eat a large dipped cone at Dairy Queen®, six doughnuts at Dunkin'Donuts®, and three large chocolate frosted brownies at the local supermarket. I'd finish the binge with a large diet soda at McDonalds®. There was little information about eating disorders over 30 years ago, but I now recognize that I was bulimic.

After all my dieting, purging, and fasting, I still graduated 20 pounds over my *original* weight (60 pounds over my lowest weight). And I had majored in the study of nutrition! Although I was certainly no role model, that first summer after graduation, I began my work as a dietitian. I was, in fact, a personal example that knowledge alone does not motivate one to change.

That summer, I got even sicker and began having what I called my "coma" dreams. Even while napping, I would fall into such a deep sleep. Although I could hear my brother or sister trying to wake me up for dinner, I couldn't move or speak. I was so scared that I was going to die, that I finally went to see a doctor. After some tests, he sent me to see a dietitian! (Mind you, I *was* a dietitian).

But that dietitian (thank you Margaret Koniz, MS, RD), helped me to recognize that when I went long periods of time without food, my blood sugar would crash to unhealthy low levels. I never told her I was bulimic, but I began to realize that the low blood sugars were what set me up to binge. Determined to stop my coma dreams, I followed her suggestions and began to eat six small meals a day. To this day, I still eat frequently throughout the day because it makes me feel more energetic. I no longer completely restrict sugar or any of the so-called *bad* foods from my eating, because I have learned that completely restricting foods only makes me crave it more.

It took years before food no longer controlled my life. And it took a few more years for me to get back to my original weight. But I wasn't binge eating, purging, or fasting. Nor was I spending every waking moment thinking about food or body fat. And that was a good feeling.

Give or take a couple of pounds, I have kept my weight down for 25 years. Whenever my weight begins to creep up, I ask myself the same questions you will ask yourself as you read this book. I have never been on another diet for I've learned that dieting only sets you up for disaster and disappointment. When I use the word "diet" in this book, I am not referring to a structured list of do's and don'ts but rather, the Webster's dictionary definition of "everything that one eats and drinks in a day."

Since my eating disorder recovery, I have completed my Masters of Science in Human Nutrition at Virginia Polytechnic Institute and my Doctorate in Adult Education at Texas A&M University focusing on personal change. For my doctoral dissertation, I studied people, who like myself, got their weight under control and kept it off. That research is the original basis for this book.

**Willpower versus SkillPower**

Take a look at your body. Do you like what you see? No? Well, then let me ask you another question: Do you know more about diet and exercise than your body shape demonstrates? It doesn't surprise me; most people do! If you're like the average American, you've already heard quite a lot about nutrition and exercise. Every magazine has a new diet. The latest diet is always a popular topic on television and radio. In fact, I wouldn't be shocked if you told me that you know so much about diet and exercise that you could write your own book!

But, if you already know what you should be doing, why aren't you doing it? Don't feel bad, you're not alone. In fact, two-thirds of all American adults are overweight; 25% are obese. This high rate of overfatness is not because Americans don't recognize that they need to lose weight. And it's not because they don't know that exercise is good and that calories count.

It all boils down to this simple fact. Research demonstrates that knowledge alone doesn't necessarily bring about corresponding changes in behavior. And yet most weight-loss programs are structured around giving you more diet and exercise information. Think about it, does simply knowing the fat content of your favorite foods make you stop enjoying it?

While we may need to bone up on our knowledge of diet and exercise in order to get the best results, that isn't what is most needed. What is lacking from those who have not been successful at permanent weight loss is the skills to get from I *know* it - to I *do* it. Notice I didn't say that the successful people have more willpower. Too often I have heard people use this as an excuse: "I just didn't have the willpower to stay with the program." It's as if they believe that willpower is something you either have or don't have.

After reviewing the research examining people who have successfully lost weight, I found that weight loss occurs only if and when an individual is ready to make changes, has decided to do it for themselves, and has empowered themselves to design their own program. The successful weight losers didn't follow any *one* specific diet and exercise program. There is *no* one perfect diet and exercise program for everyone - only the *one* that works for *you*. So don't worry about not having willpower. There are 7 distinct skills that will help you to get the results you want. These are the skills that make up *Dr Jo's No Big Deal Diet*.

This book is based on two kinds of research. First, research (including my own) that asked people who have been successful at losing weight: "How did you do it?" And secondly, research that looked at the difference between those who succeeded and those who either dropped out of programs or regained the weight. I've combined this research with more than 20 years experience counseling individuals and conducting seminars nationwide to develop this practical, hands-on program to help you learn from the successful.

**Are You Ready?**

When I first began my research, I looked at what differentiated people who were successful at losing weight from those who were not successful. I assumed I would find one diet that worked better than the rest. But when I compared the successful from the non-successful, I found there was *no* difference. For each type of approach (the same exact diet or the same exercise program), there were successful cases and those who failed. If there was no difference between the approach of these two groups, why did *some* people keep it off while *others* gained the weight back? It has to do with mastering the seven skills of *Dr Jo's No Big Deal Diet.*

Before we reveal the seven skills, it's important to find out if you're ready and committed to change. So, answer the following questions as truthfully as possible.

**√ Activity:**
Are you ready to lose weight?

1. *Why do you want to lose weight? What is your motivation? Are you doing it for you or are you losing weight to make someone else happy?*

_____

_____

_____

2. *What other major changes or adjustments are you going through in your life (such as a divorce, job change, dealing with death or illness of a close friend or family member, or working two jobs)?*

_____

_____

_____

3. *Changes in your life will often impact the important relationships you have. What kind of affect will losing weight have on your relationship with your friends, family, or significant other? How will you handle this?*

_____

_____

_____

4. *Do you ever binge on food to the point where you feel out of control and/or purge by self-induced vomiting; taking laxatives, diuretics, enemas, or other medications; fasting; or excessive exercise?*

_____

_____

_____

Your answers to the previous questions are very important. For any lifestyle change program to work, you must be ready to make the necessary changes. And you must be willing to do it for you, not just to make other people happy. Halfhearted attempts or doing it for *other* people will only lead to failure in the long run. Successive failures lower your self-confidence and self-esteem - making each future attempt progressively more difficult and less likely to be successful. Let's look at each question separately.

**Discussion:**

1. *Why do you want to lose weight? What is your motivation?*

Did you answer that you wanted to lose weight to decrease the risks of diseases including heart disease and diabetes, to make movements easier, to fit into the clothes in your closet, or to look and feel better? These are all healthy reasons to lose weight.

Be honest though. Are you losing weight to make someone else happy, to find a spouse, to be considered for a job promotion, for an upcoming wedding or a high school reunion? Each is an external event. These are not long-term reasons to lose weight. Why? When you lose weight to make other people happy or to impress other people or to make people notice you, you also set yourself up for failure. Let me offer you an example to help you understand why.

One of my patients, Lynn, weighed 267 pounds. Lynn told me that she was losing weight because she was sick and tired of job discrimination. She felt that she was continuously being passed over for job promotions because of her size. When Lynn started to lose weight, people began to notice her, including her boss. As you would expect, they often gave her encouraging praise. This additional attention only made Lynn angry and bitter. She wanted to ask: "Why didn't you pay attention to me before?" Out came the two-year-old rebel child that resides in many of us that said, "I'll show you." Lynn then ate until she put back on all the weight she had lost. Her anger and disappointment in other people resulted in an "I'll show you" self-sabotage each and every time. Lynn wasn't ready to lose weight for "Lynn."

Ultimately, you have to lose weight for you and you alone. Not just because your mother is worried about you or because your significant other nags you about your weight. Not because the high school reunion is coming up and you don't want your old friends to see you like this. You need to do it for *you*. Don't you deserve it?

On a 1996 Geraldo Rivera talk show, I watched a young overweight woman who was distraught. She wanted to lose weight because her male friends never thought of her as anything other than a pal. Richard Simmons, the weight loss guru, responded to her: "Before you can have a love affair with another person, you need to first have a love affair with yourself." I agree. We're not talking about an egotistical, selfish love for you and your needs only, but loving yourself at least as much as you love the other people in your life. When you love and respect yourself, you are far more likely to be committed to looking after your needs. Do you love and respect yourself enough to lose weight?

*2. What other major changes or adjustments are you going through in your life (such as a divorce, job change, dealing with death or illness of a close friend or family member, or working two jobs)?*

Sometimes a job change or a divorce can be an easy transition to a healthier lifestyle especially if you are leaving behind people who encouraged the unhealthier way of life. But often it means leaving behind a support system that is essential for our success. Do you have a new support system in place?

Changing the way you chose to eat, exercise, or even the way you think about your goals can be initially stressful if you try to make too many changes at one time. If you are currently going through some stressful situations, you'll need to be very realistic about your expectations.

Don't focus on revamping your diet and exercise program. Instead, attend a stress management or time management program. Handling stress in a healthier manner or managing your time more effectively will help your present situation and is bound to, indirectly, make you healthier. Sure, the weight loss will be slower, but people who have been successful at losing weight also took the changes very slowly and made only the changes that were the easiest. This, you'll discover, is what I refer to as the "No Big Deal" approach to weight loss.

*3. What kind of affect will losing weight have on your relationship with your friends, family, or significant other? Losing weight often has profound effects on every relationship - how will you handle this?*

Losing weight can have a profound effect on the dynamics of your relationship. It can mean spending more time on *your* needs and subsequently less time on *others* needs. For example, if you live with other people, they may not appreciate if you change the way you cook or the food products you buy. (Don't worry, this doesn't mean you won't be able to lose weight. It's just important to recognize these difficulties and come up with workable solutions). You may decide to eat out less often or chose foods or drinks that are considered to be less *fun* in the eyes of another person. Or perhaps you'll decide not to change your eating habits at all - and, instead, burn more calories. Will these people have a hard time accepting your time away from them when you go for a walk?

Losing weight often means that you will get more attention from other people including people of the opposite sex. Can you handle this additional attention or will you protect yourself by putting the weight back on? For some people, keeping on extra weight insulates them from unwanted attention or keeps them from addressing other issues in their life.

If you lose weight, will this additional attention make your significant other jealous? If your significant other has some added pounds, will he or she feel guilty that they too aren't losing weight? Will they sabotage you to put the weight back on so they won't feel so guilty? Or will you nag them to change as well?

It's best to think about the consequences of your weight loss prior to making these changes. Instead of using these as "excuses," be proactive. Ask yourself, "How can I best handle these possible scenarios?" You'll read more about this under *Skill #1: No More Excuses.*

*4. Do you ever binge on food to the point where you feel out of control and/or purge by self-induced vomiting; taking laxatives, diuretics, enemas, or other medications; fasting; or excessive exercise?*

If so, seek professional help because eating disorders are serious. The National Institute of Mental Health claims that five million Americans suffer from eating disorders. An estimated one thousand women die of anorexia each year (National Eating Disorder Screening Program). There was not much help available more than 30 years ago when I had an eating disorder, but there is now. Taking care of eating disorders is beyond the scope of this book. Two nonprofit organizations that can help you get started include:

National Association of Anorexia Nervosa and Associated Disorders
PO Box 7
Highland Park, Illinois 60035
(847) 831-3438
www.anad.org

The National Eating Disorders Organization
603 Stewart St., Suite 803
Seattle, WA 98101
(206) 382-3587
www.nationaleatingdisorders.org

So, is this the right time to lose weight? If it is, read on. Take it at your own pace and complete all the activities so you can find the perfect lifestyle that will help you get to and maintain your ideal weight.

If this isn't the right time, take it even slower. Go through the program slowly and thoroughly reflect on each of the activities. Many of my research subjects reported that they gathered information for years before instituting their final weight loss attempt. Not just information about calories and fat grams, but different ways to fit in exercise, and ways to change their thinking patterns. When it all came together they spoke of a light that came on in their head or they said, "It finally clicked." It was then that they actually instituted the changes.

As with any lifestyle change program, you won't succeed long term until you are ready to do it for yourself, not just for others. Prematurely jumping into another diet program, and then failing, will only further lower your self-esteem, making you far less likely to succeed in the future.

# Dr. Jo's No Big Deal Tips for Getting Starting:

1. Recognize that you *can* lose weight and keep it off. Other people have done so successfully, and so can you.

2. Don't rely on *will*power to get you to your goals. Be ready to learn and practice each of the skills that will give you *skill*power over your weight.

3. Take "ownership" of your excess weight. For whatever reason you have more weight on your body than you'd like, you're the only one who can do something about it. It's time to take personal responsibility for your actions or lack of actions.

4. Don't lose weight for other people - decide to do it for yourself. That commitment is the only way you'll be able to keep the weight off forever!

## My Notes:

Skill #1:

# No More Excuses

So you're ready to lose weight? Good for you! As I mentioned earlier, people who are successful at losing weight and keeping it off have mastered seven important skills. The first one, *No More Excuses*, states that to be successful you'll need to accept that the responsibility for success or failure falls upon you - and only you.

People who have been successful at weight loss often reported that they had undergone a psychological process of ownership. They had come to a full understanding that they alone were responsible for their weight. Ultimately, they admitted that 1) this is *my* problem and 2) only *I* can do something about *my* problem.

That doesn't mean that you can't consult with a dietitian for accurate nutrition information or join a support group to give you hints on how to handle some tough situations. But successful weight losers, before the weight came off, came to a realization that other people and situations would no longer be *excuses* for their setbacks. You can either accept some of the realities and learn to work around them or you can continue to use them as excuses. The choice is yours! But first, let's examine some of the "reasons" that you have not been successful in your past attempts to lose weight. In this next exercise, check off which reasons apply to you. Use the adjacent line to write some additional details about the difficulty.

## √ Activity:
*1. Why haven't you been successful in losing weight and keeping it off before? Check off all that apply.*

☐ Low metabolism
☐ Overweight as a child
☐ Too many other responsibilities
☐ Get bored, hungry, or stressed over the changes
☐ No time to work out
☐ Weight loss programs are expensive
☐ Marriage and/or children are "fattening"
☐ Unsupportive family
☐ Don't like "healthy" foods
☐ Don't like to exercise
☐ Eat out too often

## Discussion:
*1. Why have you not been successful in losing weight and keeping it off before?*

*Low metabolism?* If you feel that you have low metabolism, get a checkup. Often just a simple blood test is needed. If you have low thyroid, medication is available to treat the condition. The medication will probably prevent you from continuing to gain weight. But, contrary to popular belief, the medication will not make the excess weight just fall off. You will still have to lose weight the old-fashioned way - eating less than your body burns each day. In reality, however, only about three percent of the overweight people actually have a true metabolism problem.

Perhaps you don't have a thyroid condition but you feel that you are not burning calories the way others do. What can you do? Plenty! *Skill #5: Accelerate Your Metabolism*, offers many proven ways to raise your metabolism. These include weight training to build muscles that burn more calories, eating breakfast and adequate protein, and spacing out your calories throughout the day. Trust me, these techniques work. Shortly after my eating disorder recovery, I maintained my weight with just 1600 calories. Now (even though I'm 25 years older and weigh the same), I can eat about 2400 calories a day!

*Overweight as a Child?* If you think you are overweight now because you were overweight as a child, think again. Half of my research subjects said they were heavy as children and yet were still successful in losing weight and keeping it off.

*Too many other responsibilities?* If you're thinking that you have a weight problem because of your job, significant other, or family responsibilities, ask yourself if you are just using that as an excuse. Are you keeping yourself busy with other tasks and responsibilities (even complaining about other people's bad habits) just so you don't have to focus on *your* problem? Let me offer you a couple of examples.

Beverly worked full-time and had two young busy children. But she still found a way to fit in exercise. While the children were playing baseball, for instance, she would run around the field rather than sit in the bleachers. She searched for low fat meals that can be prepared quickly. If losing weight is really a priority, like anything important in your life, you will "find" the time needed.

Are you *too* involved with people in your life – and using that as an excuse? I remember once when a couple (Barbara and Jim) came into my office. Jim, a thin man, was there for dietary counseling to help lower his cholesterol while Barbara, who was very obese, accompanied him since she did the food shopping and cooking. Every time I asked Jim about what he ate, Barbara would jump right in with comments such as "I tried to prepare low fat foods like he's supposed to have, but he won't eat it. He makes me fry everything." When I asked him if he had any exercise routine, before he could open his mouth, she would spout, "I nag him about exercising all the time, but he just won't do it."

Do you see the situation as I did? Here is an example of a woman that is so involved in other people's lives that she does not seem to have time for her own issues. We all know that when other people bug us, we are less likely to want to make any changes. What if Barbara was to *not* focus directly on her husband's issues at all? What would happen if she decided to eat a healthier diet and start an exercise program - just for herself? Sure, Jim still has the option of driving to a fast food joint to get some fried sandwich or cooking up his own food, but chances are he will eat the healthier food she has prepared just because it's readily available. He may even join her when she takes a walk. Think about it - are you using other people's responsibilities as *your* excuse?

*Get bored, hungry, or stressed over the changes?* If you felt that you were not successful in keeping "on the program" because you got bored, hungry, tired, or stressed over the changes, perhaps your approach was too strict. That is a frequent mistake. Many dieters take an extreme approach which includes cutting out *all* sugar, *all* fats, *all* meat, and/or *all* white flour. These strict approaches are bound to fail, eventually! Very, very few people are able to maintain these restrictive eating habits for long term. People who were successful at losing weight in my research lost an average of just a half a pound a week. It may be a slow weight loss; but that also meant fewer changes so they could stick to it longer. We'll talk about making realistic goals in an upcoming chapter.

*No time to work out? Do* you feel that you were not successful in the past because you didn't have time to work out? So often my clients would claim this as their downfall, complaining about how long it takes to get to the health club, work out, shower, and get home. Who says that a workout has to be at a health club? A health club may be motivational for some, but if it stresses you out just to get there or you just can't find the time to go, you'll want to rethink the solution. Maybe you need to figure out how you can workout at home, lower your standards of how long a workout should be, or redefine what is "working out." Here are two examples of people who got creative to find time to exercise.

After seeing herself in a family picture, Dora, became motivated and lost 62 pounds. Dora had a lot of things working against her. She was married and had 13 children - and they all expected her to prepare their favorite traditional, Mexican-American high-fat foods every dinner. She didn't want the stress of changing how everyone ate, nor did she feel that she had the time or energy to prepare two separate meals. In addition, she lived in a neighborhood where it wasn't safe to walk to get exercise and she didn't have the money to join a health club.

How did she lose the 62 pounds? She took ownership of the problem and came up with solutions, not excuses. She only changed her way of eating at breakfast and lunch when other family members were not home - not at dinner when it would create more stress than she wanted to address. In addition, she burned extra calories by turning on the radio every evening and dancing with her younger children and grandchildren in the living room - not a structured exercise routine, just goofing around. I interviewed her seven years after her weight loss and she still danced every evening with her grandkids. This approach worked because she truly enjoyed spending time with her family.

From my experience of conducting stress management seminars, the number one complaint for most people is not having enough time. In order to make time for the important things in life, I suggest simplifying their life. This may include buying only wrinkle-resistant clothing (no ironing), wearing as little makeup as possible, or getting a simple hairdo.

At a full-day seminar, a woman came up to me after lunch and said, "I know there are hundreds of us here today and you probably don't remember me. But, this morning, I had hair past my waist. When you talked about making time for ourselves, I realized what I had to do if I was going to find time for myself. I got my hair cut over the lunch break. Frankly, I spend way more than an hour on my hair every day and I've been regretting the time for many years. My husband just loved my long hair, but it's time for a change!" Where are your priorities? Do you need to make some changes in how you structure your time?

*Weight loss programs are expensive?* Perhaps you thought you were not successful because weight loss programs cost too much or that weight loss meeting times were not compatible with your schedule. These excuses don't hold water because most of the successful weight losers lost the weight on their own (not using any special foods or programs) and found their own no-cost informal support system.

*Marriage and/or children are fattening?* I've heard people say that "once the kids are out of the house, I'll lose the extra weight." Then after the kids are out of the house, you hear other excuses such as needing to buy the fattening foods for the grandkids, or parties, or that the spouse wants to eat out more often. One of my patients, Bret, told me that he ate too many cookies, but he *had* to buy them for the kids. He returned a week later and said that he had made a commitment not to eat the cookies, and realized that the cookies were still there. He found out that *he* was the one eating most of the cookies – not the kids. So he stopped buying them.

Another woman, Sarah, had sworn off chips for many months because she couldn't just eat a few. Once she opened a large bag of chips, she would eat them all. But her mother was coming to stay with her for a couple of weeks. Sarah told me that her mother just *had* to have chips with her sandwich every day. Instead of having an argument with her mother, or buying the big bags of chips, which appeared to do her in, she chose to buy the single-sized servings of chips for her mother. She reported that she had no problems with the smaller sized bags. She opened one for her mother and that was it. No open bag - no problem!

The truth is, many people with families are still able to success-fully take off the excess weight. Your marriage and kids or grandkids only have a role in your weight problem if you let them. What excuses are you using?

*Unsupportive family?* If you feel that your family is unsupportive and is interfering with your weight loss efforts, address those issues first. Perhaps you need help being more assertive in ask-ing for support. Some, not all, of the successful weight losers did decide to change the food that everyone in the family eats. To make such a drastic change, you need to realize that not everyone will be comfortable with the decision. If you are not comfortable at expressing your needs and your personal priori-ties, chances are your family will coerce you into going back to the old menu.

We need to accept the fact that we can't force other people to change. Sometimes we have to just change our reaction to the situation. Martha told me that when she started buying lower fat foods, her family got upset. Instead of getting upset herself, she simply told them: "I do all the grocery shopping and all the cooking so you have two choices, either eat what I have prepared or buy your own foods and cook them yourself." Can you say that?

*Don't like healthy foods?* Most of us weren't born wanting the foods we now like. We developed the taste for them. The good news is, we don't have to give up all of the foods we like (we'll be talking more about this later). It may just be a matter of eating those foods less often or not changing our food and working in a bit more exercise instead. But if you do want to develop some healthy eating habits, your taste buds can learn how to like different foods. For example, it usually takes a couple of weeks for one to appreciate diet soda instead of regular or to enjoy the taste of sweetener in the coffee instead of sugar. And even if you think you don't like vegetables, I bet, if you try enough of them (and experiment with enough recipes), you'll eventually find one that you really enjoy! My family didn't like one of my favorite vegetables, yellow squash, until I cooked a low-fat version of squash casserole. Now they go for seconds!

*Don't like to exercise?* Good news! Exercise doesn't appear to be necessary to lose weight. Many people successfully take off the weight by just changing their diet. But I hope that you find some kind of movement that you do enjoy since there is a direct relationship between exercise and successfully keeping off the weight. If exercise completely turns you off, look for a *fun* activity that doesn't feel like exercise. We'll talk more about this later.

*Eat out too often?* Back in 1994 I went *"on the road"* as a professional speaker. Eating out more than 500 times a year, I found myself putting on weight for the first time since my eating disorder recovery. As a dietitian, I thought I'd been making healthy choices. But, I wasn't. After gathering nutritional information from restaurants, talking to managers and chefs about cooking methods, and actually weighing and measuring hundreds of food portions, I found the solution. And I wrote the book, *Dining*

*Lean,* to prove that it really is easy to eat healthy in restaurants - without having to limit yourself to just grilled chicken and salad.

I had clients who rationalized their behavior with the words *if only.* "*If only* I could eat that way for a few more months," "*If only* I had more time," "*If only* my husband had been more supportive," "*If only* my job didn't require me to travel so much," "*If only* I could continue to keep motivated," "... I just know that diet or exercise program would work." If the reason you keep straying from weight-loss approaches and going back to your old ways includes the words *if only,* you're not ready to accept ownership of the problem. Sometimes it is far easier to give in to these beliefs than accept what the truth is - that *you* are responsible for your own behavior. There will always be more than enough reasons not to succeed - until you decide to overcome those obstacles.

If you don't believe that you have the power within you to make the necessary changes, you tend to lose faith in yourself and look for others to do it for you. As I mentioned before, there's nothing wrong with getting advice or support from another mentor, friend, or health professional, but if you totally *buy into* one certain program or person, you probably won't succeed in losing weight and keeping it off. You are giving away the ownership that is necessary for long-term success. The only person who can make or break your plans is *you*!

## √ Activity:
*2. Rethink your "excuses" from activity #1. Are they real stumbling blocks or can you get around them?*

_____

_____

*3. Have you already begun thinking about some "no big deal" ways to change your lifestyle - and, ultimately, get your excess weight off? If so, write them down here:*

_____

_____

_____

_____

_____

_____

The bottom line for *skill #1: No More Excuses* is: "Are you willing to accept responsibility for the life you lead and make the choices you need for your success?"

# Dr. Jo's No Big Deal Tips for No More Excuses:

1. Stop making excuses about what you can't do; focus on what you *can* do.

2. Realize there's no need to change everything. Just a few simple changes, can make a big difference in your weight and well being.

# My Notes:

Dr. Jo's No Big Deal Diet

# Skill #2:

# Treat Yourself Right

It happens every year, all across the country. With the new year approaching, we tell ourselves that we are *finally* going to get in shape and lose weight. Come January first, we begin that new diet or exercise program. And then what happens? A few days, weeks, or maybe months later, we find ourselves back to square one. No willpower, you say? I don't believe so. Our lack of results comes from many things. One of the most overlooked is our personal belief system. Let me explain how and why our beliefs are so important to our success in managing our weight.

**Introduction to Beliefs**

Emerson once said, "the ancestor to any action is a thought." You may not be aware of it, but thoughts are running through your head all day long. Those thoughts come from ongoing information coming into the brain as well as our deeply entrenched beliefs. Our thoughts influence our actions which determines our results.

Step:           1                 2          3
Thoughts and Beliefs ➜ Action ➜ Result

Think about all the diets and programs you've been on. Did you spend most of your time and effort focusing on changing your *usual* habits by eating different foods, eating slower, eating less, and/or exercising more? Most people do. And to some extent working on your actions *can* change some of your beliefs about yourself - that's why part of the book will focus on healthy actions. But more often, these actions tend to be the motivating force that lead you to sabotage yourself. How? If deep down inside you believe that you are incapable, undeserving, or unworthy of having a lean body but go through all the motions of a low fat, healthy diet, you'll eventually fail as this example shows.

Belief:                  Action:      Result:
"I have no choice but to be fat" ➜ Eat too much ➜ Fat body

I've heard many people say, "My grandmother is overweight, my mother is overweight, my sisters are overweight. I'm going to *try* to lose weight, but it's probably senseless because of this strong hereditary trend. But I'm going to try anyway."

It doesn't even matter what the actual truth is in this situation. If you *believe* that you will be unable to lose weight, your actions will flow in the direction of this inability - and you won't lose weight. Someday, some way, you will break down. Let's just say you've already committed yourself to a diet and tell yourself that you won't have any desserts. But you end up eating one small cookie. In actuality, it's really no big deal - just 50-100 calories.

The destruction comes right after. You start berating yourself with thoughts including, "I'll never be able to lose weight. I can't stick to a program. I'll always be fat." With thoughts like that, you'll probably end up eating even more or finishing off the whole box! The self-fulfilling prophecy will always come through: "Whether you think you can or you can't, you're right!"

So instead of spending time reading up which diets the celebrities are on, buying a health club membership when you didn't take advantage of the last one, or berating yourself for always failing at diets, take a look at your beliefs about yourself, your excess weight, and your perceived ability to change by considering the following questions.

### √ Activity:
Be honest with yourself as you consider the following.

*1. Describe yourself in detail.*

_____

_____

*2. Who's happier - thin people or overweight people - and why?*

_____

_____

*3. Is being lean or overweight determined more by genetics or personal habits?*

_____

_____

*4. How do you think losing weight will change you and your circumstances?*

_____

_____

*5. Losing weight involves changing habits. Do you consider the time and effort involved to be a selfish act or one of self-love? What do your close friends and family think?*

_____

_____

*6. Is there some aspect of your excess weight that makes you feel safe?*

_____

_____

_____

## Discussion:

*1. Describe yourself in detail:*
Did you write just about your physical attributes? Women tend to think of their beauty (or lack of) as just skin deep, whereas men tend to have a healthier, more holistic attitude. If you tend to think of beauty as just skin-deep, this can greatly affect your self-esteem and, subsequently, your whole attitude about your weight. Other than physical beauty, what other attributes do you have that make you a beautiful person (such as personality traits, talents, and hobbies)?

Instead of berating yourself about one perceived weakness (overweight), consider all your positive traits. Why is this so important? When you feel good about yourself, in general, you tend to live a healthier life. Molly, with a lot of weight to lose, told me that it was difficult to look at herself and not feel depressed. She felt that it was still very important to have something pretty on the outside. So she started getting professional manicures - that way she could always look down and see her pretty hands while she worked on losing weight.

*2. Who's happier - thin people or overweight people - and why?*
If you had no idea of how to answer this question, go to a public place and take some time to watch people closely. Based on their looks alone, take some guesses about their personalities.

What are your perceptions, beliefs, and feelings about thin people? Do you have any negative beliefs about thin people that are significant enough to keep you fat? If you believed deep down inside that thin people are selfish, self-centered, narcissistic, and egotistical, your body would want to protect you from having this "terrible" transformation happen to you.

What are your perceptions, beliefs, and feelings about overweight people? Do you think of them as loving, fun, happy-go-lucky, get-along kind of people? Do you see how dangerous any of these generalizations can be to your attempts at weight loss? Do you worry that losing weight will make you less liked by others? Remind yourself that being thin or overweight doesn't automatically determine your personality traits. Be open to seeing the exceptions to your negative beliefs.

*3. Is being lean or overweight determined more by genetics or personal habits?* Research says both are involved. But your answer establishes your core belief about your ability to change. If you believe that you're destined to be overweight because of family tendencies, then you will probably not be successful at weight loss until you change those beliefs.

Genetic tendencies can be very strong in determining your weight. But, be honest. Did your genes make you overweight or did you just *inherit* some bad habits including poor food choices and a tendency to be sedentary? If your entire family is heavy going back many generations, your chances of becoming a *Twiggy* may be slim. But that doesn't mean you can't get down to a healthier weight.

People who have been successful at weight loss described a set of skills that helped them lose the weight. But *all* learned skills still need to be practiced to keep them sharp. A concert pianist doesn't become great and then stop practicing, and expect to stay at the top. Sure, there are a few naturally lean people who have good genes and don't have to even think about maintaining a healthy weight. But, I think if you ask around, you'll find that most lean individuals have just practiced these healthy habits until they became second nature.

*4. How do you think losing weight will change you and your circumstances?* Do you think being leaner will make you happier? While losing weight on the outside may make you look different, losing weight alone doesn't make *you* different.

One of the reasons why people lose weight and then put the weight right back on is because their life *doesn't* change. They lose weight and expect their whole life to change – find the perfect love, the perfect job, etc. When it doesn't they say "Oh well, what difference does it make." And then they gain all the weight back. Now do you see why it's important to lose the weight just for yourself?

*5. Losing weight involves changing habits. Do you consider the time and effort involved to be a selfish act or one of self-love? What do your close friends and family think?*
Many people, especially women, are taught early in life to focus all of their time and attention on other people in their life. Remember Barbara and Jim from the previous chapter? Although Jim came to see me for dietary counseling for his high cholesterol, it was Barbara that needed some serious help with her weight.

While she knew that eating healthy would be good for both of them, she said she couldn't adhere to a healthy diet since she *has* to cook for her husband - and that he doesn't want to eat healthy. If you believe taking care of *yourself* is much lower on the scale of importance than taking care of everyone else, you'll never succeed. Ask yourself: aren't you *just as* important as the other people in your life? Remember what Richard Simmons said, "before you can have a love affair with another person, you need to first have a love affair with yourself."

*6. Is there some aspect of your excess weight that makes you feel safe?*
Is it somewhat scary to think of having a lean body? Some people's self-esteem is so low, they actually feel unworthy of having a body of which to be proud of. What are your beliefs regarding having a lean body? Do you think that other people's reactions and expec-

tations of you would change? Do you worry about how to handle any extra attention you might get? Do you think that other people may expect more from you at home and at work? Sometimes keeping on extra weight helps to keep you from addressing these and other related issues in your life.

Sue found that each time she lost weight, her husband paid more attention to her - attention with which she was uncomfortable. So she found herself gaining the weight back so that she could get back to the comfortable relationship they had before.

Lynn, gained more than 100 pounds after a date rape. While not on a conscious level, her weight served as her protection. Can you understand why she found it difficult to lose the weight? Luckily, she got some psychological counseling to help her to understand that the rape was not her fault and to change her beliefs about her weight.

Do you see how important it is to look closely at your beliefs? Your beliefs can be so strong that they can help to sabotage your actions - or they can positively move you in the desired direction. Remember, "whether you think you can or you can't, you're right."

**How To Change Your Beliefs**

If you believe you are unworthy of losing weight or unwilling to deal with both the positive and negative consequences of losing weight, then all your thoughts and actions will work against you - and you will fail. As we mentioned earlier, eventually, you will find yourself in situations where you end up sabotaging yourself. You will also fail if you expect your life to dramatically change or if your fat is protecting you from some real or imagined consequence.

On the other hand, if your healthy actions are in accordance with your healthy beliefs, the effort will be easier. It was Rene Descartes who said, "I think, therefore I am."

41

## Dr. Jo's No Big Deal Diet

Do you need to change some of your beliefs? Here are four ways to change your unhealthy beliefs into beliefs that serve your goals:

1. Practice the "No Big Deal" approach
2. Decrease your negative self-talk
3. Increase your positive self-talk
4. Visualize your success

### 1. Practice Dr. Jo's "No Big Deal" approach

It is possible to have good self-esteem or feel very competent in one area of your life and not in another. Sometimes it is frustrating to know that you have been successful in your chosen career or are a great parent or have other fine successes, but have failed in the area of weight loss.

Results from research state that people will only continue on a weight loss plan if they are concerned with their health or appearance *and* if they believe they are capable of changing. Your belief in your capability is based upon your *perception* and not necessarily your true capabilities. It shouldn't surprise you that the more diets you have been on and failed, the less likely you are to believe that you can actually make a successful change.

We'll discuss how to alter your perception of your ability to change, but first, let's talk about a frequent reason we fail in our attempts to lose weight. So often it is because we go to extremes in our attempts. We give up *all* of our favorite foods, spend a great deal of time preparing new foods, and tell ourselves that we must exercise *every* day. As soon as we don't follow through completely on our "perfectionistic" (and unrealistic) rules, we tell ourselves we are failures, trash the whole program, and go back to our old ways. No wonder we have a difficult time believing that we will be able to keep up a program for a long time or forever.

It's only natural that we tend to cling to the familiar things in our life. The habits we have, even if they are not the healthiest, are comfortable. So any change takes away some of our sense of security. The more drastic the change, the less likely we will be successful at keeping it up. How much change can you handle before you go back to your old, comfortable ways?

The people who were successful at losing weight and keeping it off made only small changes in their diet and exercise routine. True, they didn't lose weight quickly - only an average of a half a pound a week. But they were able to keep it off! (Think about this. If you began losing a half a pound a week just a year earlier, you'd now be 26 pounds lighter!) For their final attempt at weight loss, the successful decided that they were not working on a "diet" but rather a lifestyle change designed to make their life easier and more comfortable in the long run.

If you introduce a change into your life that you think of as a burden, it *will be* a burden. To increase the belief in yourself to succeed, think about making small, incremental changes that would be "No Big Deal" to implement.

Now you see why my patients called this the "No Big Deal" approach to weight loss. Over and over again, I'd hear them say, "Oh, that's no big deal. I can do that." Each small, easy step can be readily accomplished to give you a sense of achievement with little stress. With each boost of confidence, you'll be ready to add additional small changes to achieve the results you desire. Because the changes are so small, you'll be far more likely to succeed. Let me offer you an example of a person who made just *one* "No Big Deal" change that made a *huge* difference.

Mark was a police officer in Houston. On the hot days (and, in Houston, there are many), he would drink at least six large cola drinks from fast food restaurants. When he switched to diet sodas (and made no other dietary or exercise changes) he lost 87 pounds over the next year!

**Here are some additional "No Big Deal" ideas:**
- always leave at least one bite of food on your plate
- jump on a mini-trampoline during television commercials
- replace dessert with fruit one night a week
- add a 10 minute walk every day
- replace one unhealthy snack with a healthier one
- play catch with the kids instead of watching television
- go out to lunch every other day rather than every day
- ask for the restaurant to serve dressing, sauces, and toppings on the side - so you can control the amounts used
- replace your high calorie chip with a lower fat, baked chip
- use less oil in your favorite recipe
- add more vegetables (and less meat) to your evening meal
- switch from whole milk to 2% low fat (or skim) milk
- take the stairs instead of the elevator
- walk briskly instead of strolling

Remember, there's is no need to make *all* of these changes. Think about instituting just one or two of the No Big Deal changes at a time! The list was just some of the ideas, what others can you think of?

**√ Activity:**
*7. "No Big Deal" ideas that I will use include:*

_____

_____

_____

## 2. Stop negative self-talk.

The second way to change your beliefs is to stop your negative self-talk. Most of us are unaware of the thoughts that constantly run through our head. Listen in and, chances are, you'll hear evidence of damaging self-talk. You call yourself names, scold yourself, and blow things way out of proportion. And then instead of feeling positive about changes you make, you use the word *"trying"* to demonstrate to yourself how unsure you are of yourself.

How often do you tell friends that you're "trying" to lose weight? You're either working in that direction or not. In order to stop negative self-talk, it's important to keep the following things in mind.

♦ **Don't call yourself names**

When you trip over a door frame or chair leg, what do you say to yourself? Do any of these sound familiar: "I'm a klutz. I'm always tripping over things. Way to go, Grace! Oh goodness, I wonder who was looking?" When your mouth runneth over and you say something that you realize soon after was not the best words to use, what do you say to yourself? "Why can't I keep my big mouth shut? That was a stupid thing to say. There I go again, I blew it!"

What do you say about your body? Do you ever call yourself names? "Fatso? Thunderthighs? Jelly Belly?" What do you say when you bite into one of your "forbidden foods," the food you said you would *never* eat for the rest of your life? Do you call yourself a pig? When filling out a nutrition form for me, a patient named Frank once wrote, "Fat Frank," where his name should have been.

If you were overweight as a child, you undoubtedly remember the hurt you felt when someone called you names or sang songs such as, "Tubby, tubby, two feet wide." Perhaps you were not overweight as a child but you remember other negative names you earned because of real or imagined attributes. I was called "red-headed freckle-faced monkey." Back then, the name only made me hate my bright red hair more.

Do you really think any of this insulting language motivates you? (Think about it. What's the best way to motivate children? By putting them down with insults? Of course not! Children are best motivated with a positive approach - and so are we.) Names hurt and degrade our self-esteem. And the lower our self-esteem gets, the more likely we are to continue with unhealthy behaviors. It's a vicious cycle. As an adult, chances are other people no longer call you names. But are you continuing to call *yourself* names?

## √ Activity:

*8. What names do you call yourself?*

_____

_____

_____

### ◆ Don't scold yourself

Do you yell at yourself for not having any self-control? Do you hang up all your dieting efforts with a statement such as "Well, I blew it! Might as well eat the rest of the bag"? We don't just say it to ourselves. I've heard people make personal jokes about themselves when they are with a group of people, such as "I have no willpower" or "I'm going to regret this when I get on the scale" when they order dessert.

Have you ever scolded yourself with "shoulds" such as "I should have exercised this morning" or "I shouldn't have eaten that?" Most of the time it's about situations that are over and done - something you can't do anything about. Stop "should-ing" on yourself!

Chances are you have heard parental advice that you should never say to a child: "You are a bad girl" or "You are a bad boy." Although we don't always make the best choices, no one person is completely bad. Instead parents are advised to tell their children that the specific *behavior* is bad. If only we could remember that advice for ourselves!

## √ Activity:

*9. What negative things do you say to yourself or aloud? Do you ever scold yourself?*_____

_____

_____

## ♦ Don't blow events out of proportion

Another part of negative self-talk is blowing events out of proportion. These include lines like: "I really blew it," "I was so bad," "I binged," or "I pigged out." If you hear yourself start to talk like that, examine the reality. People often start in with the statement: "I really blew it," long before they really do. They eat one cookie or one chip and they tell themselves they "blew it," and the negative self-talk is what leads them to really blowing it. One cookie or chip is not "blowing it."

As a counselor for many years, I have heard the confession "I was *so* bad" hundreds of times. When I asked my client to tell me why they were bad, they describe a situation where they perhaps didn't make the wisest choice, but it wasn't really "so bad." And, besides, even a poor decision does not make them *bad* people.

## √ Activity:

*10. Do you ever blow events out of proportion? If so, what do you say?*

_____

_____

_____

## ♦ Don't use the word "trying"

Saying that you are *trying* to lose weight is another self-fulfilling prophecy. Think about it, you don't usually say that you are *trying* to eat four candy bars. You either ate four candy bars or you didn't. There is also no such thing as "trying to lose weight." So either say that you are making healthy changes or you are not - but not that you're *trying*.

## √ Activity:

*11. Do you use the word "trying" when talking about losing weight? Rewrite what you could say instead.*

_____

_____

_____

When you say negative things to yourself such as: "Here you go again. You have absolutely no self-control. You're a failure" - you will be! Would you use this type of language with your friends? Of course not! And would you let your friends talk to you in this fashion? I hope not. So start treating yourself with the same love and respect; stop the negative self talk right now!

### 3. Use positive self-talk on a regular basis.

The third way to change your beliefs is to use positive self-talk. Positive self-talk can be instituted in two ways to help you achieve results with your weight loss plan. First, you'll want to use positive self-talk to replace your negative self-talk. Secondly, use positive self-talk statements throughout the day to increase your confidence.

Think about a recent compliment you were given. Didn't it make you feel good? Instead of waiting for others to reinforce your beliefs about yourself, your body, and your ability to sustain your desired changes, give yourself compliments in the form of positive self-talk throughout the day. Positive self-talk doesn't have to be just about eating or exercising. Use positive self-talk to remind yourself that you are a person and not just a weight. You consist of your whole entity including your personality and all your strengths and talents. If you can't think of any positive things to say to yourself, think about what your friends and mentors would say to you.

Each time you catch yourself saying something negative, break the chain by saying "stop, stop, stop." Then say something positive and proactive.

♦ **Use positive self-talk to replace the negative self-talk:**

| Instead of: | Say: |
|---|---|
| "I've got a party to go to today; I'm going to blow it!" | "I enjoy feeling in control when I go to parties." |
| "Oooh, that looks so good." | "I'm tempted to eat this but it's more important to be lean." |
| "It's Christmas (or their birthday, or my anniversary) so I've got to eat it." | "I can enjoy these foods anytime I want and I chose not to eat them right now." |
| "Well, I just ate those cookies that I said I wasn't going to eat. I'm going to eat the whole bag eventually, so I might as well finish the whole bag off right now." | The few cookies I just ate won't make me fat. It's over and done and I'll stop right here." |
| "I can't believe it. I've been watching what I've been eating and I still gained a pound!" | "I'm making wise choices. This weight gain is just temporary. I am confident that my weight will go back down." |
| "I've only lost a half a pound." | "I just lost two sticks of butter off my hips." |
| "I shouldn't have eaten that. I can't stick to anything." | "It's over; it's done. What have I learned so this doesn't happen again?" |

# Dr. Jo's No Big Deal Diet

## √ Activity:

12. *When you hear your negative self-talk, ask yourself what your best friend, mentor, or counselor would have said to you if you had spoken those thoughts aloud - and make revisions. Write down some things you have said in the past and then write a more positive comment to use in the future.*

| Previous Comments: | Revised Comments: |
|---|---|
|  |  |
|  |  |
|  |  |

♦ **Use positive self-talk (affirmations) throughout the day to reinforce your efforts:**

When you look at the positive self-talk examples that follow, you may instinctively laugh and say "Oh, I can't say that. It's not true." If you do, I have two suggestions. First, find one you *can* believe in. Secondly, remember "any lie can be believed if it's simply repeated often enough." Following are some examples of positive affirmations.

• "I enjoy eating low fat foods."
• "I am working on healthy eating habits."
• "I am a person of great value at all times."
• "I enjoy feeling in control."
• "I love to exercise. It feels good to move my body."
• "I (your name), am a thin person, I stop eating when I am not hungry, and I weigh (desired weight) pounds."
• "I love myself unconditionally."
• "I am strong, confident, and successful."

√ **Activity:**

*13. Write several positive self-talk statements or affirmations to practice throughout the day:*

_____

_____

_____

## 4. Visualize Your Success

Do you know how to worry? Most of us do - and we do it well! What is worrying? It's when you dwell on a situation and only think about the worst possible scenarios. If you know how to worry, then you can easily learn how to visualize. Visualization, another powerful way to change your beliefs, is just the opposite of worrying. You see yourself dealing with a situation and succeeding. Although visualization requires repetition and practice, it's as simple to do as day dreaming.

Visualization is nothing new for athletes. It is currently used by nearly every professional sport team as well as with Olympic teams. Sports psychologists assist the team members to see, within their "mind's eye," themselves succeeding within their sports - successfully shooting baskets, skating the routine perfectly, or running faster than they had ever before. How does visualization work?

Dr. Peter Fox at the University of Texas Health Science Center/San Antonio conducted research on the powerful effects of visualization. In several experiments, he attached brain electrodes to athletes to measure their brain activity. He found regardless of whether they were imagining themselves participating in a sports event or really practicing the activity, the same parts of the brain were stimulated.

In many regards, the brain can't tell the difference between a real event and an imaged event. Don't believe it? Have you ever watched a scary movie (which you *know* isn't real) and still jumped during the scary scenes? When you worry (about something which hasn't even happened) do your muscles get all tight and your stomach upset? Of course! These examples show us that our thoughts really do influence our body's reactions.

We can use visualization to our benefit. The more we do something, the more confident we'll be that we can do it again. This is really no different than an actress or actor rehearsing their lines over and over again (whether in their head or outloud) until they can perform their part without much thought. When you want to learn a new skill, use visualization.

## √ Activity:

*Several times a day, close your eyes and relax. Imagine yourself with a lean body and watch how it moves and how it feels. Doesn't it feel good? To get that body, you'll want to develop some healthy habits. Some of these don't come second nature. Picture yourself handling one of these situation the way you want to. For example, if it's difficult to control your food intake in restaurants, imagine yourself taking a slice of bread and then pushing the bread basket to the other side of the table, asking for the doggie bag when you order your meal, and leaving a small amount of food on the plate. You may also want to practice turning down seconds at your next dinner party or handling that nasty comment that a family member always makes. Visualize every detail of the environment and practice your lines. Visualize those difficult situations over and over until you believe that you can handle them.*

*14. I will practice visualizing these situations for the following results:*

_____
_____
_____

Don't worry if you don't believe everything that you tell yourself with positive self-talk or everything you see with your visualization practices. You may not, at least in the beginning. But eventually your mind will begin to believe what you are feeding it and your actions will go in the direction to support your self-talk and visualizations.

**Live Your Life Now**

Have you allowed your weight to put your life on hold? Overweight people often put off going to the beach, the gym, the singles group, or on a trip until they lose weight. Successful weight losers found that when they started living their life once again, they felt better about themselves, and, thus, strengthened their *Skill*Power to "stick with it." The following visualization exercise will help you get in touch with what you may be missing in your life.

## √ Activity:

*Pick a quiet time in the day. Close your eyes and relax. Imagine that you have the most incredible metabolism - no matter what you eat, you won't ever gain an ounce! You are now at your ideal body weight. Picture yourself with the body you would like to have. Look at your legs, your abdomen, your chest, your arms, your face. Then ask yourself the following questions and brainstorm for a minute or two before jotting down your thoughts.*

15. *If you had the perfect body and the perfect metabolism, how would your life be different?*

_____

_____

16. *If you had the perfect body and the perfect metabolism, what kind of person would you be?*

_____

_____

_____

17. *If you had the perfect body and the perfect metabolism, what would you eat and when?*

_____

_____

_____

*18. If you had the perfect body and the perfect metabolism, what would you be doing differently?*

_____

_____

_____

**Discussion:**
For successful weight loss, you'll want to start thinking, moving, and acting like the thin person inside of you. Start living life rather than just watching it pass you by.

*15. If you had the perfect body and the perfect metabolism, how would your life be different?*
*16. What kind of person would you be?*

Did you imagine you and your life to be quite a bit different than they are today? Would you be more outgoing and fun-loving? Getting more attention from others? Is this realistic to expect? What if you expect your whole life to change when you lose weight and it doesn't? That disappointment may make you stray from your weight loss plans. Ask yourself, why aren't you the person you imagined yourself to be? Why isn't your life as much fun as you want it to be? Why can't you be that person right now in your present body? What's holding you back?

*17. What would you eat and when?*
I'm not suggesting that you really *will* be able to eat everything that you visualized whenever you want and in whatever quantity you want. But this exercise helps you to realize what foods or styles of eating really appeal to you. It will be important to utilize this knowledge into your plan for success. You'll discover later in this workbook, that allowing yourself to eat the foods you love will help you to stay on your plan.

*18. What would you be doing differently?*
What did you picture yourself doing in the previous exercise? These are the things that make you good. Don't wait until your weight comes off - do it now!

People who have been successful at weight loss often said that they started to live in the present. They didn't wait to have fun or to be fun people until the weight came off. Start having fun now while you wait for your body to catch up.

**√ Activity:**
*19. What will you do now, not later to live your life to its fullest?*

_____

_____

_____


**Love Yourself**

Some people feel guilty about spending time and effort on themselves because they feel that their family, job, friends, or professional organizations need them more. They tend to say *yes* to everyone but themselves. As Steven Covey states in his book *Seven Habits of Highly Effective People*, we must take care of ourselves before we can adequately take care of the others.

People who have been successful at losing weight tell researchers that they began to spend more time on themselves - not in a selfish way, but in an act of self-love. I'm not suggesting that we love ourselves to the exclusion of other people. I want you to spend *as much time* on yourself as you spend on *other* people. When we do things that support the lean person inside us, we feel better about ourselves, and others tend to have more respect for us as well.

So, every day do something just for you. Establish habits that treat you as if you count - and don't feel guilty!

# Dr. Jo's No Big Deal Diet

Here are some ideas:
- get the sleep you need even if the house is messy
- read a book for pleasure
- eat breakfast every day, even if it's a quick bagel and a banana on the run.
- fit in a daily walk or bubblebath - whatever makes you feel good
- prepare the foods you love, instead of always catering to others' desires
- go rollarblading, play on the swings
- work on your photo album, needlepoint, or paint
- go for a drive in the country, hike in the woods, or play in the ocean
- buy yourself fresh flowers
- get a massage, manicure, or pedicure on a regular basis
- drink a cup of tea by the fireplace or by candlelight
- watch a movie without feeling the need to fold clothes, iron, etc.

## √ Activity:
*20. What will you do just for you?*_____
_____
_____


In the Introduction we discussed how it was important to be ready for change. *Skill #1: No More Excuses* encouraged you to take responsibility for your actions instead of blaming others - and focusing on what you can do, rather than focusing on what you can't. *Skill #2: Treat Yourself Right* helped you to work on building a strong belief system to support your actions and start loving the whole person that you are. In the next chapter, we'll examine the rules of your plan.

# Dr. Jo's No Big Deal Tips for Treating Yourself Right:

1. Examine your beliefs. Are there any that are preventing you from reaching your goals?

2. Work on changing your beliefs before you change your diet or any other part of your lifestyle.

3. Practice the *Dr. Jo's No Big Deal* approach by making small, achievable goals rather than setting yourself up for failure.

4. Listen to your self-talk. Focus on correcting the negative self-talk to reflect the true picture and practice positive self-talk to help you to achieve your goals.

5. Practice visualization to help you get through difficult situations.

6. Start living your life now rather than waiting until you are thin. It can be as simple as taking a few minutes everyday just for you.

# My Notes:

Skill #3:
# Make Your Own Rules

Most weight-loss programs, whether it is an expensive, structured program or one straight out of a magazine or book, dictates what you should do. Designed by true (or self-proclaimed) experts, they tell us exactly what to eat, what to drink, how much and when. In addition, they often tell us how to exercise, how much to exercise, and when to exercise.

This "one-size-fits-all" approach teaches us to listen, not to ourselves, but to an *external* person or program that takes the control, the rules, and the success for the entire process out of our hands. And strangely, we often love it!

As a counselor, I don't know how many times I have heard - "Just tell me what to eat and I'll eat it." "If you tell me I need to exercise, then I'll do it." Many of us ask to be taken by the hand and led down the road to success. It sounds easy, but unfortunately, this structured plan will probably backfire at some point.

Why? There are at least three reasons. First of all, many of us still have that two-year-old rebel child within us. Think about what happens when we demand that a typical two-year-old do something? Just by nature, he or she often does just the opposite. When someone or some program is dictating *our* life, that two-year-old rebel inside us comes out and, with an I'll-show-you attitude, sabotages our efforts. This is true even when we've asked these people to change our lives.

Another reason why structured programs fail is that we learn to distrust our own judgment. The control we give to other people (and weight loss programs in general) undermines our confidence that we are in control of our weight. That's why if we just break the rules ever so slightly, we feel as if we have *blown it*. Then we feel guilty of our failure and we *"hang it up."*

Thirdly, many of us are able to eat what someone tells us to for awhile but eventually we bore of the same old foods and miss our favorite ones. But chances are, the program didn't include these favorite foods so, we didn't learn how to moderate our intake. When we do have our favorite food, we tend to overeat it. It's no surprise that people drop out of diet programs because they begin to miss their favorite foods, their usual pattern of eating, and other aspects of their lifestyle that was changed.

During my research study, I queried my study participants about their "secret" diet for success. Their answer? One woman summed it up when she said, "it's not the diet you choose but rather how you view the rules." In other words, there's no reason to cheat provided *you* set the rules, rather than someone else. Many of them expressed the change in their mindset from being on a "diet" to making healthy lifestyle changes. And we also know that like most things in life, one program can not fit all. It must be individualized.

*Dr Jo's No Big Deal Diet* approach to weight loss is similar to what a good psychologist or counselor does. A good counselor doesn't tell you what to do. They listen, ask appropriate questions to get you to think, perhaps give you some ideas, and then help you come up with the answers that are best for *you*.

The secret program to help you lose your excess weight is within you right now. The only way you will be successful (long-term) is to honestly listen to yourself, become your own authority, and make our *own* rules - ones you can stick with long-term. This chapter is all about designing your own program for success.

**Have a Plan**

As I've mentioned, people who have been successful at losing weight and keeping it off did not follow any one particular weight-loss program. Instead they designed their own plan for success. They thought about what had worked and what hadn't and learned from both their successes *and* failures. This helped them to realize what was important to them and how much change they were capable of. To help you design your program for success, complete the following exercise regarding all of your previous attempts to lose weight.

**√ Activity:**
*1. Think of all the ways you previously lost weight and write them down on the following chart. Keep these things in mind:*

• Approaches -
  Write down each diet/exercise program you've used. The names of the diets or exercise programs are not as important as are the details of what was encouraged or restricted. Examples of diets include: high protein, fasting, kept fat grams under 20g, vegetarian.... Instead of just writing *exercise*, write specifics including the type of exercise, frequency, and length of time.

# Dr. Jo's No Big Deal Diet

- Why did you stop -
  List the major reason(s) why you stopped each of the approaches you mentioned in the first column. Reasons may include: the program was too expensive, you didn't feel well, you were always hungry, you couldn't make the meetings, took up too much time, got bored, food variety was too limited, or had reached your goal...

- Advantages -
  Spell out what worked with each of your approaches. This may include things such as easy to do, wasn't hungry, enjoyed the exercise, lots of choices, lots of energy, lost weight quickly, good tasting food, meetings at convenient times, motivational leader, liked the individual attention, included foods I like....

- Disadvantages -
  Spell out the disadvantages (the things that you didn't like) about each of your approaches. This may include things such as difficult to adhere to, always hungry, didn't like the exercise, limited food choices, low energy level, no/little weight loss, food didn't taste good, meetings not at convenient times, didn't like the leader, limited food choices, don't like working in groups, not enough support, took too long to prepare the food ...

| Approaches Used | Why Stopped? | Advantages | Disadvantages |
|---|---|---|---|
| | | | |
| | | | |
| | | | |
| | | | |

# Dr. Jo's No Big Deal Diet

## √ Activity:

*2. Looking over the previous chart, summarize below what you perceived to be the advantages and disadvantages of the programs you've been on or other ones that you've considered. (There are no right or wrong answers). Consider describing the following in your list:*

- *Meals - best number of meals to eat, time to eat, types of foods to include, whether to include pre-prepared/ convenience/ frozen/ packaged foods, how often to go to restaurants...*
- *Record keeping - keep track of foods eaten/ quantities/ calories/ fat, etc. or not?*
- *Snacks - needed or not, what types of snacks, time to eat them*
- *Support - best to lose weight on your own/ with a partner/ in a group, people who help/ hurt you in your effort, other tools to use...*
- *Exercise - type, length of time, frequency...*
- *Special occasions - what works for birthdays, holidays, office parties...*
- *Evaluation of success - how to measure success: scale, energy level, food records, blood sugar levels...*

*Advantages (things that appeared to work for you)*

_____
_____
_____
_____
_____
_____

*Disadvantages (things that don't work for you)*

_____
_____
_____
_____
_____
_____

### Learn From Your Mistakes

You may have found some contradictions, but it's crucial to work at least some of the advantages into your final weight-loss plan. While it's important to look at what worked with each of the previous weight-loss attempts, it's just as critical to learn from your mistakes. Henry Ford once said "A failure is an opportunity to begin again more intelligently." Take a close look at everything that didn't work, ask yourself why, and then figure what you can learn from it. It's important that you interpret it correctly. The following are some illustrations of how to make your program more successful by including things that work for you.

| Initial Analysis | More In-depth Analysis | Possible Solutions |
|---|---|---|
| Low calorie frozen meals are boring | It wasn't really the low calorie meal that was boring. I miss the companionship of my coworkers who eat out every day. And I like getting out of the office. | • Learn how to order low calorie selections in my favorite restaurants<br>• Try to get some of my coworkers to eat in with me. After lunch, go for a walk outside<br>• Eat my frozen meal at the local park<br>• Eat out just three times a week instead of every day |
| It's hard to stay on any program because my family likes junk food. I have a hard time staying away from those foods. | I buy those foods for them because I don't want them to feel deprived. | • Talk to the family. Ask them to hide the junk food so I don't see it and get tempted<br>• Buy these foods in single-serving packages; they're less tempting<br>• Give my children money to buy the junk at school so I don't have to bring it home |

| Initial Analysis | More In-depth Analysis | Possible Solutions |
|---|---|---|
| Joining a program where food was provided sounded easy, but it didn't taste good. | I need the support of a group, but I don't like having to eat only their food. | • Find another program that has better tasting food or allows me to buy only some of the food<br>• Learn how to modify my favorite home recipes to make them lower in fat and calories; join a support group that doesn't require me to buy their food |
| I thought joining a health club close to work would be motivational but I still don't feel like working out. | Joining a health club close to work may have been a noble idea, but I'm too hungry to go there after work. | • Work out at lunchtime or before work<br>• Bring a snack to eat before I work out<br>• Eat my larger meal at lunch rather than dinner<br>• Join a health club closer to home<br>• Forget the health club and buy some workout equipment for home |
| I can only stick to a program Monday through Friday – weekends are impossible. | I starve myself to death during the week – no wonder I'm hungry all weekend. Plus I eat more on the weekends because I'm bored. | • Plan to eat more during the week, especially snacks that keep my energy up during the day<br>• Find friends to have fun with on the weekends – may a ski club<br>• Get back into fishing – I miss it plus I can't eat while I'm handling bait |

Those are just some examples of how to work around a few sticky situations. Skill #3 is all about designing your own program for success so the correct solutions are up to you.

## √ Activity:

*3. Take a look at some of your difficult situations and come up with two or three possible solutions.*

| Initial Analysis | More In-Depth Analysis | Possible Solutions |
|---|---|---|
|  |  |  |
|  |  |  |
|  |  |  |

## Redefine "Successful" Weight Loss

Turn back to the first exercise at the beginning of this chapter. Put a star next to the weight loss program that was your best approach. Why do you consider it your *best*? Most people mention the program that allowed them to lose weight fast or had quick results. You may also have selected the program that was easy to follow, mindless, made you feel good, or gave you lots of energy. The real question is: did this approach also give you the tools you needed to *keep* the weight off?

Chronic dieters often think only about how they can *lose* weight. I've heard people say, "If only I can lose weight I *know* I'll be able to keep it off!" In reality, research (and perhaps your past experience as well) doesn't back this statement up. How many times have you lost weight, and then not kept it off?

When we get in shape, most of us recognize that simply getting to the "fit" stage will not keep us there. We need to exercise on a regular basis in order to keep that fit shape. This is no different than the continuous training and practice that a surgeon, scientist, or professional athlete undergoes throughout their career. They need to practice the skills to keep them sharp.

Therefore, we need to change our paradigm of *successful* weight loss to include both losing the weight *and* keeping it off. Successful programs are those that not only bring about weight loss, but also provides you the skills you need to keep the weight off - forever!

Years ago, I had a patient named Ray. When attempting to work on his personal plan for success, he suggested that he would like to go on a fast (have only water and juice) to get the weight off. He said, "that's the only way I lose any weight." I asked him how many times he has fasted ("dozens of times"), how much weight he lost ("as much as 30 pounds"), and how fast the weight came back on ("often twice as fast as it was to lose it"). Finally, he realized his distorted thinking. A quick weight-loss approach that always results in the weight returning is *not* successful. Always judge a *successful* weight loss approach on whether it helps you to lose weight *and* keep it off.

Do you think that keeping the weight off is more difficult than losing weight? From personal experience you might think this is true. But keeping the weight off doesn't have to be so difficult. People who have been successful at weight loss reported that when they made only small changes in their life and lost the weight slowly, keeping the weight off was easier because healthy lifestyle patterns were already established.

No doubt, it does take time to do this analysis and to work on your action plan. But by examining the advantages and disadvantages of your programs of the past, you will be on your way to formulating your personal program for success - *your* secret formula. Isn't this better than spinning your wheels over and over again?

I did the following exercise many years ago. At that time I was still involved in my bulimia. I was either on a very low calorie diet, bingeing on thousands of calories, or fasting to try to burn off the extra calories of the binge. I finally realized that when I cut my food portions drastically or skipped meals, I tended to overeat at some point in the near future, often leading to a binge. Eating three meals a day wasn't even enough for me, my body wanted food six times (or more) a day. Everything that I had read on dieting suggested that eating between meals was only adding unwanted calories and contributing to my problem. But, I decided to trust myself rather than some diet "expert" and found success. When I ate smaller portions of food every three hours I felt more in control, did not binge, and eventually lost the unwanted weight. Forever! Nearly 30 years later, I still eat every three hours.

Carl told me that he always started his weight loss program by promising to exercise an hour *every* day. While it always worked to get off the excess weight, eventually because of family or work demands, he would get out of the habit. And shortly afterwards, he'd be off the program. He finally realized that some exercise was better than none and shifted his plan to include at least fifteen minutes, five times a week. Although he could do more (and often did), he was almost always successful in meeting his goal - and was able to stay with it.

Another patient of mine, Paula, told me that she had read that sugar was evil. She was convinced that sugar was the sole source of her low energy and weight gain. So she got rid of all the sugar. Paula not only cut out the candy, cookies, and soda but searched for no-sugar salad dressings, bread, and crackers and the like. On top of that, she had read an email about the dangers of artificial sweeteners, so she omitted all of the sugar-free foods containing aspartame, saccharin, etc.

It probably wouldn't surprise you if I told you that she couldn't stick to the program very long, but that she *still* kept going back to the same strict rules over and over again. I suggested that she take her plan one step at a time. She decided to use the artificial sweeteners as substitutes for now (the email she received was a hoax - check out www.snopes.com). Paula realized that avoiding sugar was easy during the work week, but it was more difficult during the weekend. So she decided to let herself have her favorite sweet on the weekends in limited amounts. That plan was more manageable - and it worked long-term.

The third skill of *Make Your Own Rules* suggests that you look at the way you set up the rules of your personal weight-loss program. Non-flexible rules are precursors for failure. As soon as you make one tiny slip, you feel like a failure and go off your program completely.

√ **Activity:**
*4. Considering long-term success rather than just losing weight, what considerations do you think will help you to be most successful?*

_____

_____

_____

_____

This is a good exercise to do with close friends or in a weight management group. If the group is empowered to challenge each other's perceptions, the insight and perspective of others will help to see the situation more clearly. After you've come up with a few ideas, try out your plan. If it works, great! But if some part of it doesn't work, ask yourself why it didn't. Then keep revising it. Continually be open to new ideas. If something isn't working, don't just scrap it. Instead, ask yourself what can you learn.

**Set Realistic Goals**

Most people measure their progress by their weight loss but are unrealistic about how fast they should be able to lose weight. When these unrealistic expectations are not met, they have a tendency to throw in the towel! So let's address setting realistic goals by answering the following questions:

♦ **Setting Weight Loss Goals**
√ **Activity:**
*5. What is your ideal weight?* _____

*6. How fast have you been able to lose weight in the past?*

_____

*7. How fast do you think you should be able to lose weight?*

_____

## Discussion:

*5. What is your ideal weight?*
There are plenty of charts out there. I purposely did not include one because you've probably seen them all. Instead of going with a chart, ask yourself what weight you feel good at and can realistically achieve and keep long-term. If you have a lot of weight to lose and have no idea of an achievable goal, keep the goals more achievable - starting with an initial goal of just 10 or 15 pounds.

Don't forget to establish a *realistic* weight goal. Once, when I was training for both a triathalon and a marathon, I got about ten pounds lighter and it felt great. But this weight wasn't realistic unless I wanted to work out two times a day for the rest of my life (and I didn't) or closely monitor my food intake (which led to constant hunger).

*6. How fast can you lose weight?*
All of us have had different experiences regarding weight loss. Some of us remember when we dropped a quick five or ten pounds in just a week or two. Others have stayed on a program and were frustrated because they lost nothing. What has been your average weight loss per week or month in your past?

*7. How fast should you be able to lose weight?*
Many people think that they *should be able* to lose weight quickly, but that is often unrealistic. We forget that our excess weight didn't come on overnight and won't come off that fast either. How fast *you* should be able to lose weight, is dependent upon how many calories you need to maintain your weight in the first place.

While some of us have better metabolisms that others, generally speaking, the number of calories we need to maintain our weight is determined by what we weigh, the composition of our weight (muscle vs. fat), and how much energy we expend with our movements and exercise.

Generally speaking, the more you weigh, the more calories you need to maintain that weight. Therefore, as you lose weight, your body needs fewer calories. That's why we can lose weight for weeks or months and then reach a plateau. So plan, as you lose weight, to readjust your mindset about how much you can eat. Fortunately, our hunger will also adjust at the same time so we won't want to eat as much.

Men can often eat more than women and lose weight faster than women because they generally weigh more and have a greater muscle mass (muscles burn more calories than fat). While active men have about 12-15% body fat composition, active women have 18-22% body fat. This fact is also one of the reasons why we all burn fewer calories as we age even if we weigh exactly the same. As we get older, we tend to be less active and, thus, have a lower muscle percentage which means we burn fewer calories.

Here's a two step process to find out how fast you can realistically lose weight.

**Step one:**
Although there is some variation (based on genetics and the variables just discussed), you can estimate your daily calorie needs using the worksheet below.

### Estimating Daily Calorie Needs

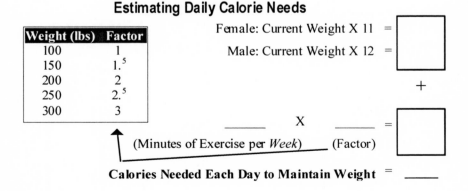

| Weight (lbs) | Factor |
|---|---|
| 100 | 1 |
| 150 | 1.$^5$ |
| 200 | 2 |
| 250 | 2.$^5$ |
| 300 | 3 |

Female: Current Weight X 11 =

Male: Current Weight X 12 =

+

_____ X _____ =

(Minutes of Exercise per *Week*) ___ (Factor)

**Calories Needed Each Day to Maintain Weight** = _____

Once you know approximately how many calories you need every day to *maintain* your current weight, you can estimate how fast you can lose your excess weight. Since there are approximately 3500 calories in one pound of fat, you must eat 3500 calories fewer calories than you need - to lose one pound. How fast you can lose a pound depends on how quickly you can decrease your calorie intake or increase your activity level.

> **3500 calories = 1 pound of fat**
> **(looks like 4 sticks of butter)**

**Step two:**
An easy way to calculate your expected weight loss is to subtract 500 calories a day (3500 calories divided by 7 days in a week) for each pound a week you would like to lose. For example, if you need 1500 calories a day to *maintain* your current weight, cutting back to 1000 calories/day can realistically result in just one pound a week weight loss.

| Maintenance Calories Per Day | | Expected Weight Loss |
|---|---|---|
| 1500 calories | - 500 = 1000 calories/day<br>- 1000 = 500 calories/day<br>- 1500 = 0 calories/day | 1 pound/week<br>2 pounds/week<br>3 pounds/week |

Of course, this is just a rough estimate. The real question is could you eat *just* 1000 calories per day on a long-term basis? Probably not.

I've heard clients scold themselves because they didn't lose the four or five pounds that week like they expected. They tell themselves they were "bad" because they didn't reach their goal. I hope you now realize that, for most of us, it is *impossible* to lose four or five pounds in a week. For those people who have experienced a four to five pound drop in a week, it's important to realize that most of the weight is not coming from fat. It is coming from water. For example, high protein diets cause an unnatural diuretic response leading to a large water loss in the first few weeks. Since a healthy body is about 60% water (and higher if you have a lot of muscles), the body replaces it as soon as the person goes back to a mixed diet.

How fast can *you* lose weight? In the first column, fill in your maintenance calories (from step one). Then follow the formula to calculate the number of calories you'd need to consume to lose one, two, and three pounds per week.

| Maintenance Calories Per Day | | Expected Weight Loss |
|---|---|---|
| _____ calories | - 500 = _____ calories/day<br>- 1000 = _____ calories/day<br>- 1500 = _____ calories/day | 1 pound/week<br>2 pounds/week<br>3 pounds/week |

Be honest, which of these levels are realistic for you to follow on a longterm basis?

Experts suggest that we attempt to lose no more than one or two pounds a week. There are at least four reasons: 1) the just-mentioned calculation shows it's almost always physically impossible, 2) it's difficult to get adequate essential nutrients in under 1200 calories, 3) a rapid weight loss causes a loss in lean muscle mass which can lower your metabolism, and 4) rigid dietary and exercise changes are difficult to maintain. Remember, also, people who have been successful have lost weight even slower - averaging just a half a pound a week!

## ◆ Setting Goals other than Weight

As mentioned earlier, using weight as a goal is only one way to structure a program. And it's probably not the best since we don't always have control over it. Weight can fluctuate, as much as ten pounds during a month, even if we eat the same thing every day. And besides, since muscles weigh more than fat, we can actually get thinner without taking off weight.

Instead of weight goals, it's healthier to set realistic *behavior* goals that spell out exactly what you plan on doing. Since you can not control other people's behaviors, be sure the focus is on what *you* will do. With our busy life, it is easy to get sidetracked from our good efforts without specific, written goals. Goals, which are not specific and realistic, are just dreams.

The following offers, first, some examples of some unrealistic and then some more realistic goals. Then there are some vague and then more specific goals.

| Instead of: | Make the goal more *realistic*: |
| --- | --- |
| I will never eat desserts or sweets or anything with sugar. | I will eat my usual dessert five times a week (instead of daily) and have fruit on the other two evenings. |
| I won't eat out. | I will eat out once a week. I will call the restaurant ahead of time and ask the manager for some suggestions on managing my calories and fat needs. |

| Instead of: | Make the goal more *specific:* |
|---|---|
| I will lose 55 pounds by Dec. 31. | I will lose ½ pound a week by switching to skim milk, walking 10 minutes 5 evenings a week, eating out just once a week… |
| I will eat fewer than 1200 calories per day. | I will eat a breakfast of cereal and skim milk, snack only on fruits, … |
| When Mom tells me to take the rest of dessert home with me, I will tell her that it is her fault that I am overweight. | When Mom suggests I take the rest of the dessert home with me I will say, "No thanks Mom, I'd rather not." |
| I will work out more often. | I will walk the dog for 10 minutes while dinner is cooking. |
| I'm not going to berate myself. | When I catch my scolding myself about the one cookie I ate, I will say, "Stop, stop, stop. That was just one cookie. It's OK. I'm still on the program." |

Keep in mind that these suggestions are not necessarily what you *should* be doing. These are just ideas to get you started. You and only you can make up the rules for your "No Big Deal" approach to weight control.

# Dr. Jo's No Big Deal Diet

## √ Activity:

*8. Set at least three specific, realistic goals (other than weight). Like the examples above, describe what you will do and not what you will be. Make them specific and realistic.*

Goal #1:_____

_____

Goal #2: _____

_____

Goal #3: _____

_____

There's an old Chinese proverb that says "a journey of a thousand miles begins with but a single step." As you can see, it isn't willpower that makes the difference between success and failure. The secret involves making small, realistic, achievable changes in your life that over time sustains a weight loss. Having written goals can make that difference. Be sure to review and update your goals regularly because life keeps changing.

# Dr. Jo's No Big Deal Tips for Making Your Own Rules

1. Don't buy into a weight loss program lock, stock, and barrel. Make up your own rules based on what works for *you.*

2. Be creative when looking for solutions of things that hinder your progress.

3. Redefine a successful program as one that will not just bring about a weight loss, but will help you keep it off.

4. Set realistic weight-loss goals of no more than two pounds a week. Keep in mind that successful weight losers averaged a half pound a week.

5. More important than weight-loss goals are behavior goals. These should focus on specific, achievable things that you will change in your behavior.

# My Notes:

Skill #4:

# No More Deprivation

Any lifestyle change can be stressful. It only makes sense that bigger changes bring about more stress than smaller ones. The people who were successful at weight loss and long-term maintenance made only modest (and reasonable) changes in their lifestyle.

Throughout this book, you have been developing your plan for successful weight loss. Many times, I've mentioned the importance of making small "No Big Deal" changes in the way you think and act so you don't feel deprived.

There are three additional ways to not feel deprived. First, I encourage you to cut back only slightly on your usual food intake - think of developing a healthy lifestyle that will lead to a healthy weight. Second, listen to and feed your hunger - you *can* relearn this ability you had when you were young. And lastly, include your favorite foods into your life plan. I know what you're thinking - "I can't control myself with those foods." But let me ask you, although you undoubtedly do lose weight when you avoid all your favorite foods, are you able to stick with the program for very long? Probably not. Most people can't give up their favorite foods indefinitely. And that's OK, because you don't have to. Most successful dieters reported that their programs did not deprive them of their favorite foods. You *can* re-learn how to eat with satisfaction without gorgeing.

## Be Calorie Conscious

If you look on the bookstore shelves, you'll find lots of diet books that guarantee success. Dr. Atkins claims that you can eat all the protein and fat you want and still lose weight. Since there are only three nutrients that contain calories (protein, carbohydrate, and fat), this high protein/high fat diet is very low in carbohydrates.

Dr. Dean Ornish's diet, on the other extreme, cuts out animal protein and most of the fat. He says a diet rich in carbohydrates is the secret. In the middle of the debate are recommendations set by the American Heart Association, the American Cancer Society, and the American Dietetic Association. Each of these groups recommend a moderate protein/moderate fat diet that is focused on carbohydrates – but not nearly as high as Dr. Ornish's approach. Who's right?

### ♦ Limit your calories to less than you currently burn

At the March 2000 National Nutrition Debate, it became quite clear that *any* diet (if adhered to) works to take weight off. The secret is not whether you cut back on proteins, fats, or carbohydrates. Since the only nutrients that contain calories are proteins, carbohydrates, and fats – cutting back on *any* of these nutrients will reduce your total calorie consumption. Eating fewer calories than you burn is the ultimate secret to weight loss!

But to keep it off successfully, you may need an approach that is not far different than the way you currently eat. Successful dieters lost weight using a variety of eating plans, but most tended to fall into a more moderate approach. So the question is not which diet is best, but rather which diet is best for *you*. There is not *one* diet that fits all. The perfect plan for *you* will fit your food preferences, eating style, personality, and lifestyle.

There are many ways to eat fewer calories. Here are some suggestions:

• Make a few "No Big Deal" changes - Eat and drink what you are now, with a few, small changes. For example, switch to diet soda instead of regular, eat 2 cookies instead of three, or use lowfat cheese instead of regular. It doesn't sound like much, but every little bit counts!

• Think value - When you go shopping for groceries, clothes, or a car, do you look at the price? Sure! Why? Because you want to see if you can afford it or if it has or exceeds the value of its price tag. In addition to not having a limitless bank account, we also do not have a limitless calorie need. So try this same approach with food. Become aware of the calories you are eating by reading labels. Then, before eating it, simply ask yourself, "Is it worth $x$ calories?" For example, I like onion rings. But when I found out each one has 100 calories I decided that they were just not worth it! (On the other hand, chocolate chip icecream *is* worth 300 calories a scoop!)

• Keep a food diary - Write down everything you eat and drink. That's it! As simplistic as this advice is, it works for many people because it makes eating a more conscious activity.

• Count calories - Write down everything you eat and drink, calculate the calories of each, and keep your calories under the total number that you determined from the previous chapter.

• Follow a calorie plan - Set up a meal plan allowing yourself a specific number of calories at each meal.

• Follow a structured meal plan - Instead of focusing on calories, allow yourself a predetermined amount of specific types of food at each meal (Find a Registered Dietitian to help you at www.eatright.org).

- Make it simple - Some people have been successful by making very simple rules they could live by. For example, "don't go back for seconds," "only fruit after dinner," or "don't skip meals."
- Add more exercise - Don't change your eating habits at all. Instead focus on adding more exercise into your life.

## √ Activity:

1. *Which method(s) to cut calories are you planning to use?:*_____

_____

_____

♦ **Cut no more than 500 calories from your maintenance calories**

If you've decided that you need to count calories to be successful, how many fewer calories? Refer back to the previous chapter when you calculated how your maintenance calories and estimated your weight loss at three different levels.

Planning a weight loss of a pound a week (or cutting 500 calories from your maintenance calories) is a good place to start. If you have a tendency to binge eat, perhaps start with a cut of just 100-200 calories. Getting too hungry will only set you up for another binge.

## √ Activity:

2. *If you've chosen to count calories, what number is appropriate to promote a slow (but permanent) weight loss:*_____

_____

♦ **Keep your fat grams under 30% of your total calories**
Now that I've said that it doesn't matter whether you cut back on carbohydrates, proteins, or fats, I also need to remind you that heart disease is the number one killer in the United States. In addition to being overweight, eating a diet high in cholesterol and saturated fats often raises your serum cholesterol, one of the risk factors for heart disease. So, if you love meats and fats, you still may want to cut back to stay healthy. And for you carbohydrate-lovers who try desperately to stick to a no- or low-carbohydrate diet (which is high in fat), do you really want to go the rest of your life without baked potatoes, bread, corn, popcorn, fruits, and other foods high in carbohydrates - especially when there's no need to suffer?

Many researchers report that simply lowering your fat intake will stimulate a faster weight loss. That's because while proteins and carbohydrates have four calories per gram weight, fats contain *nine*. That's more than twice the calories for the same weight amount. Research has also shown that while extra calories in the form of fat are easily converted into body fat, extra carbohydrates are not. When you eat 100 calories of carbohydrate more than your body needs, 23 calories are wasted in the process of changing it into body fat - only 77 calories are stored! So, extra fat calories are really about *three times* more caloric than extra carbohydrate calories.

Cutting back on fat also appears to be helpful because fat calories are more dense. Choosing more carbohydrates and less fat means that we can eat more food. Picture five cups of air-popped popcorn, two cups of watermelon, or a thick slice of freshly baked bread. Each food has 100 calories. On the other hand, there's also 100 calories in just a tablespoon of butter!

As you can see, if you like eating a substantial amount of food, cutting back on the fat is helpful. If you can enjoy that "fried" egg cooked in a nonstick skillet with dry toast, you'll easily save 100

85

calories without leaving any food off your plate. But this simplistic advice can be misleading and disheartening for many people working towards weight loss if they eat *too much* of the low-fat foods.

The advice to simply cut back on fat worked a generation ago when few *processed* fat-free foods existed. Today there are literally *thousands* of lowfat and fat-free foods including low fat Twinkies®, Snack Well® cookies, baked chips, and fat-free frozen yogurt. And many of these highly processed foods have just as many calories as the original. Remember that it's still the calories that count. Eating an extra 3500 calories of *fat-free* calories will still result in one pound weight gain of *fat.* So if simply counting fat grams works for you, go ahead and do it. But for those of you who have a hearty appetite and tend to overeat the fat-free foods, that alone may not do the trick.

If you agree that you should cut back on fat, how low do you want to go? While Dr. Dean Ornish and others suggest cutting fat intake back to 10% of total calories, most people can't tolerate this vegetarian, *no* added fat approach to living. Could you?

The *average* American is eating about 34% of total calories in the form of fat (which means half of all Americans are eating *more*). The American Heart Association, American Diabetes Association, and the American Cancer Society recommend a fat intake of 25-35% of total calories. And, research shows that most people who have lost weight and kept it off longterm eat somewhere between 20 and 30% of total calories in fat. Could this level be achievable for you? Take a look at the following chart to see what your fat "budget" would be.

**30% Fat Budget**

| Calories | 30% Fat (gms) |
| --- | --- |
| 1200 | 40 |
| 1500 | 50 |
| 1800 | 60 |
| 2000 | 67 |
| 2500 | 83 |
| 3000 | 100 |
| 3500 | 117 |

Then compare that number to the food labels or get a book that lists fat grams. One of my other books, *Dining Lean*, is a good reference for those who eat out. It lists calories and fat grams of most menu items in every type of restaurant.

There are some diets that suggest that you can lose weight simply by calculating the percentage of fat in each individual food and avoiding any food that has more than 30% of their calories coming from fat. If you're interested you can calculate the percent of fat using the following formula.

**How to calculate the percentage of fat in a food item:**
   1. Grams of fat X 9 = _____ (# of Fat Calories)

   2. _____ divided by the Total Calories = _____

   3. _____ X 100 = _____ % Fat

This simplistic rule, by itself, doesn't always allow you to lose weight. Using this guideline, the program would allow you to eat as much lollipops, fat-free yogurt, or fat-free cookies as you want since they're all 0% fat. But if you're likely to overeat these foods, you won't lose any weight. As I just mentioned, extra calories (even if they are fat-free) will still make you fat.

This type of plan also unnecessarily restricts the foods you *can* eat. Does it make sense to outlaw oil (100% fat) completely at any amount and then allow a pancakes that have oil in the recipe but whose final product is only 10% fat?

In addition, some foods have very little fat, but because the calories are also low, the fat percentage is high. Low fat salad dressing is an example. If a tablespoon of salad dressing has 10 calories and 1 gram of fat, then 90% of the calories are coming from fat (1 gram fat X 9 = 9 calories from fat/10 = 90% fat). Doesn't it seem silly to eliminate low fat salad dressing just to avoid one gram of fat?

Calculating the percentage of fat is good to know if you want to assess if a product is as lean as its description suggests. For example, "2% lowfat milk" suggests a very low fat product, but it isn't. The "2%" is not a calculation of the percent of fat but rather describes that 2% of the *weight* of the milk is coming from fat. From looking at the label you find that one cup of 2% milk has 150 calories and 5 grams of fat - and has 38% of it's calories coming from fat!

Percentage of fat in 2% Low Fat Milk:
1. <u>5</u> grams X 9 = <u>45</u> calories coming from Fat
2. <u>45</u> fat calories/<u>150</u> total calories = <u>.38</u>
3. <u>.38</u> X 100 = <u>38%</u> Fat

If you're curious, whole milk contains just 3½% of the total *weight* from fat, but about 48% of the total *calories*.

On the food label you will also find the "% Daily Value." This is not the same as the percentage of fat calories. Percent of Daily Value is based on the percentage of calories in a standard 2000 calorie diet. If you are eating 2000 calories a day, you can use these numbers to add each of the "% Daily Value" and stop when you get to 100%. Unfortunately, if you are eating less (or more) than 2000 calories, this number can be misleading.

Although you *can* add up % Daily Value, you can not add up the calculated fat percentages. Nor can you simply average the fat percentages. Just because you eat one food at 10%, another at 20% and a third at 30% - you can't assume the average is 20% - it depends on the total calories of each of the products. Now you see why I recommend that you simply add up the grams of fat of each item and compare it to your needs in the chart on the previous page - it's so much easier.

### ◆ It's the Little Things that Count!

In discussing the "No Big Deal" approach to weight loss, I mentioned that every little change could make a BIG difference over the long run. Let me show you how. Based on the scientific fact that there are 3500 calories in a pound of fat, just 10 extra calories per day will add up to an extra pound of fat accumulated each year. That 10-calorie difference is why the average American gains an extra pound a year after the age of 35!

$$3500 \text{ calories} = 1 \text{ pound fat}$$

| If each day you eat an extra: | You would gain this much weight in a year: |
|:---:|:---:|
| 10 calories | 1 |
| 100 calories | 10 |

Cindi came to see me after gaining 15 pounds over the previous nine months. She swore she had developed a metabolism problem because "I haven't been doing anything different." But three endocrinologists confirmed that everything was normal. After I reviewed everything that she ate and drank, she began to realize that the weight gain was completely accounted for by a slight change in how she "decorated" her coffee.

She drank four big mugs of coffee a day, putting two tablespoons of creamer in each mug. That adds up to a half cup of creamer each day (2 tbsp X 4). Originally, she was drinking Creamora® but nine months earlier she had switched to International Delight Creamer®. She inadvertently added an extra 180 calories each day explaining nearly all of the 15-pound weight gain:

$$\frac{1}{2} \text{ c. International Delight®} = 360 \text{ calories}$$
$$\frac{1}{2} \text{ c. Creamora®} = \underline{180} \text{ calories}$$
$$180 \text{ calories/day extra}$$

$$180 \text{ calories/day X } 30 = 5400 \text{ calories extra/month}$$

$$5400 \text{ calories/month X } 9 = 48{,}600 \text{ extra calories}$$
consumed over 9 months

$$48{,}600 \text{ calories/3500 calories in a pound} = 13.9 \text{ pounds!}$$

Another client, Jill, got concerned about the safety of sugar substitutes after reading an internet chain letter. So she switched from two *diet* sodas a day to two *regular* soda pops and promptly gained 10 pounds over a four-month period. The weight gain is easy to explain once you understand that while all sodas are fat-free, two cans of regular sodas contain 300 calories. Multiply that 300 calories by 120 days (four months) and you see that it adds up to an extra 36,000 calories or 10 extra pounds (36,000/3500 calories in a pound).

As I mentioned earlier, the email chain letter about the dangers of aspartame, is a hoax. Research evidence confirms that sugar substitutes in moderation are safe. I personally, don't worry what dangers moderate amounts of non-nutritive sweeteners may pose. Obesity and the increased risk of heart disease, high blood pressure, and diabetes are real, known risks. And if using sugar substitutes helps you to cut back on the calories, go ahead and used them moderately. If you are greatly concerned about the safety of these products, make it a goal to cut back *after* the weight has come down.

Here are just some of the possible small changes that can make a big difference over time. Don't institute every one of these ideas at the same time. Think about these as possible goals for the future.

## How to Save 100 Calories (or more) a Day:

- Eat fresh fruit instead of juice - chances are you will eat less because fresh fruit is more filling (and juice has just as many calories as soda)
- Have an English muffin or bagel instead of a biscuit or croissant
- Try egg substitutes instead of eggs scrambled (and in your favorite cookie recipe and in the French toast)
- Use lowfat cheese in the lasagna or grilled cheese sandwiches
- Switch from a large cup of whole milk to skim
- Use skim milk instead of creamer in your 4 cups of coffee
- Ask for the small fries instead of the medium with your burger meal
- Switch from regular soda to diet soda
- Order your sandwich without cheese
- Use mustard instead of mayo on your sandwich
- Take one tablespoon of butter off your baked potato
- Leave the extra butter off the movie popcorn
- Try a lowfat frozen yogurt instead of ice cream
- Order the luncheon portion at dinner - many restaurants allow this even if it's not on the menu (savings are often hundreds of calories)
- Ask for the salad dressing on the side - dip your fork into the dressing and then into the salad for a taste with every bite
- Order grilled fish and chicken instead of fried
- Remove the skin off the chicken
- Order your favorite pasta dish with tomato sauce instead of cream sauce - or ask for *half* the cream sauce
- Don't just get steamed vegetables - order them "steamed without butter"
- Ask for your stirfry to be prepared with less oil
- Have your bread without the butter

- Use a non-stick spray to grill the pork chops and use it on the airpopped popcorn, too
- Skip the cheese sauce on your broccoli
- Switch from granola to wheat flakes
- Scrape the icing off the cake
- Make a fruit smoothie instead of an icecream milkshake

The important thing is to cut back where it is "No Big Deal." Every little calorie adds up. Keep in mind that some people will call you picky because of your preferences. Remind yourself that you're being picky about the body you wear - and that's OK.

## √ Activity:

*3. What small changes can you make (diet or exercise) that would make a BIG difference over time?* _____

_____

_____

_____

## Feed Your Hunger

You have probably heard that you should eat only when you are hungry and stop eating when you are full. That's easier said than done because this advice is so subjective. One way to make your hunger level more objective is to use numbers to illustrate how full or hungry you feel.

The hunger scale, as shown on the next page, ranges from zero to 10. Zero is when you are feeling *starved to death* whereas ten is feeling *stuffed like a turkey*. Five is halfway in the middle - feeling comfortable.

## Hunger Scale

| 0 | 1 | 2 | 3 | 4 | 5 | 6 | 7 | 8 | 9 | 10 |
|---|---|---|---|---|---|---|---|---|---|---|
| Starved | | | | | OK | | | | | Stuffed |
| to death | | | | | | | | | | like a turkey |

The advice to "eat only when you are hungry" could be disastrous if you tend to overeat when you are *too* hungry. I found out years ago that when I hit a 0 or even a 1 on the hunger scale – look out! I would eat everything in sight! After some tests, I found out that my blood sugar drops very low three hours after a meal and I get shaky, grumpy, and weak. Does that happen to you? Perhaps, instead of waiting until you hit rock bottom, you might want to eat when you reach a two or even a three on the scale.

Should you stop eating when you feel full? It depends on what you mean by full. Some people have mentioned that they rarely feel full. But perhaps you can remember a past Thanksgiving (or other special day) meal you really overdid it and you felt bad. That's a number 10. You definitely want to stop before you reach a 10. But when?

I like to think of five on the scale as feeling OK - neither hungry nor feeling full. Perhaps you want to stop eating at five or six. Be realistic. None of us likes to feel hungry yet we want to avoid stuffing ourselves too often. If you find yourself stuffing yourself on a regular basis, it's important to look at other issues in your life. We'll discuss this more in skill #6 *Ask Yourself Why*. If you currently eat to a 10 every day, cutting back to a nine is still realistic – and will help you to lose weight.

## √ Activity:

*4. Think about when you are not on a diet. How do you typically eat at your biggest meal of the day? Circle the number at which you typically start and stop eating.*

**Hunger Scale**

| 0 | 1 | 2 | 3 | 4 | 5 | 6 | 7 | 8 | 9 | 10 |
|---|---|---|---|---|---|---|---|---|---|---|
| Starved to death | | | | | OK | | | | | Stuffed like a turkey |

Considering what you know about when you typically start and stop eating, think about when you *plan* to start and stop eating. If you tend to overeat when you get *too* hungry, you may need start eat at an earlier time when your hunger is not so high. Or you may choose to eat more often throughout the day. Keep track of your hunger scale for awhile and then make the appropriate adjustments in when and how often you eat.

## √ Activity:

*5. Circle the number at which you plan to start and stop your eating at a meal:*

**Hunger Scale**

| 0 | 1 | 2 | 3 | 4 | 5 | 6 | 7 | 8 | 9 | 10 |
|---|---|---|---|---|---|---|---|---|---|---|
| Starved to death | | | | | OK | | | | | Stuffed like a turkey |

Keep in mind that thirst often imitates hunger. So letting yourself get thirsty may make you more likely to overeat. Drink at least 8 cups of water a day to prevent this problem. An easy way to meet your water quota is to keep a large drinking bottle of water with you at all times. Sipping it throughout the day is easier than forcing yourself to drink a cup at a time.

For those of you who don't like water, add a lemon or lime wedge to the water or drink mineral water. You can also get the water your body needs from a non-caloric, no-caffeine drink such as decaffeinated coffee, tea, or diet soda. Other products include sugar-free Koolaid®, Crystal Light®, or non-caffeinated, flavored waters containing 0-10 calories per serving. A few cups of caffeinated beverages a day are generally considered safe.

√ **Activity:**

6. *Do you drink enough water or other non-caloric, no-caffeine beverages?*_____

7. *How can you increase your water intake?*_____

_____

## Eat Your Pleasers, Skip Your Teasers

A sure way to fail at your weight loss approach is to eliminate all of your favorite foods from your plan. Why? First, you'll miss them because they taste good. Your favorite foods also have strong emotional, social, and cultural ties for you as well. Your preferences may bring back special memories and the feelings associated with them. Thirdly, there's no reason to deprive yourself.

The solution is to learn how to eat them in moderation, not to exclude them completely. This may be true even if you tend to overeat these particular foods. Later we'll discuss how to keep from overeating, but first let's find out what your favorite foods are.

♦ **Eat your pleasers**
Your first indication may have been from our imagery activity from Skill #2. These may be foods we like to reward ourselves with. Some favorite foods are tied into holidays, birthdays, end of the week, or other celebrations. What are some of your favorite foods. And, don't say "everything." What would you choose to

eat if it were your last meal? Did you think about just general groups of foods such as fried foods, sweets, or salty foods? Candy? Or ice cream? That's a start, but I want you to think in even more detail. For example, think about what type, brand, and other qualities. Instead of listing just "cookies," perhaps what you really love are your Mom's homemade butter cookies. Instead of ice cream, could it be a rich chocolate chip ice cream that has chocolate chips of a certain size? You may like fried foods, but perhaps very hot French fries from Burger King® are your favorite. If you think you are not that picky, think again. It's important to narrow down our favorites into just a few. I call these foods your "pleasers."

## √ Activity:

*8. List your pleasers and the reason they are your favorites.*

| Favorite Foods | Reasons Why? |
|---|---|
|  |  |

To be successful, don't deprive yourself of your pleasers. Plan on treating yourself every now and again - how often is up to you. It may have to be less often or in smaller quantities than you typically eat them, but not so infrequently that you feel deprived.

Do you have a difficult time controlling how much you eat of your pleasers? Here are some proven tips:

- Don't deprive yourself. Bingeing is often the result of what I refer to as the "last supper syndrome." That's when you tell yourself that this is the last time you can have it ever.
- Be discriminating. Eat only the very best quality. Don't settle for anything less. If it's not great, tell yourself you'll wait for the best!
- Eat it slowly and enjoy every bite without feeling guilty.
- Enjoy your pleasers while dining out in a restaurant. It's difficult to ask for seconds and the rest of the cake or pie isn't sitting around your house to haunt you. It also reinforces that eating pleasurable foods doesn't have to enjoyed in secret.

#### ◆ Skip your teasers

Don't get your *pleasers* confused with your *teasers*. Teasers are foods which are convenient, easy to get, look better than they taste, or aren't on our mind until we see it. These may be food that we currently eat and perhaps overeat, but they are not necessarily our favorites.

Teasers may be the candies you eat each time you pass the candy bowl on your secretary's desk or at the bank counter. It may be the open bag of chips that taunts you to reach in for a handful each time you pass the kitchen. Or your mother's pie that you don't really like, but don't want to hurt her feelings. The clear difference between the pleasers and the teasers is that if you had a choice, you would pick the pleasers.

**√ Activity:**

*9. Name your Teasers and describe where and when you eat them:*

_____

_____

_____

_____

_____

_____

_____

If you still don't have a lot of detail about your pleasers, try this next activity.

**√ Activity:**

*10. Sit alone in a quiet place with your favorite foods. Pick up the food and smell it. Does it smell good? Feel it with your fingers. Take a bite. Roll it around in your mouth and truly taste it. Is it sweet? Salty? Gritty? Crunchy? What qualities do you perceive? Is it at good as you expected it to be? We all have to make choices, so ask yourself, "Is it worth the calories?"*

Alice Jo did this exercise and narrowed down her "pleasers" to a special brand of imported chocolate and her mother's oatmeal cookies. Now she doesn't eat just any chocolate, she waits until she can get across town to get the brand she really wants. Then she buys just a couple of ounces and savors every bite. She doesn't buy storebrand cookies anymore because she realizes that they don't "please" her the same way as homemade oatmeal cookies. So she waits until she goes to her mother's house to get what she *really* wants.

## √ Activity:

*11. Now come up with a plan to eliminate many of the teasers that you currently eat. These might include not buying them, having an honest discussion with others about having these teasers available, bringing your own snacks so these teasers aren't so attractive, or making sure you don't get too hungry and give in. You decide how you can best handle the situations.*

_____

_____

_____

_____

_____

_____

_____

Skill #4 is about removing the feelings of deprivation from your lifestyle plan. If you pay attention to your hunger level and focus on your Pleasers rather than your Teasers, you'll find yourself losing weight while enjoying the foods you love.

# Dr. Jo's "No Big Deal" Tips for No More Deprivation

1. Eat fewer calories than you burn by making small changes in the way you eat.

2. Listen to your hunger. Eat when you're hungry and stop before you are too full.

3. Give yourself permission to eat your pleasers (your favorite foods). It'll make it so much easier to skip your teasers.

## My Notes:

# Skill #5:
# Accelerate Your Metabolism

Would you like to be able to eat more food without gaining weight? You can - by increasing your metabolism, the rate in which your body burns calories. You can accelerate your metabolism by moving your body more, eating breakfast, and spacing your calories throughout the day.

**Move Your Body**

While successful dieters didn't always use exercise in the weight loss process, nearly all felt that physical activity was important in keeping the weight off. Not only does exercise burn calories, building muscles help you to burn calories at a faster rate - 24 hours a day!

Don't like exercise? Maybe you just haven't found the right exercise for you. Exercise isn't just running or doing an aerobics class. Other forms of movement can include yoga, gardening, dancing to MTV, and actively playing with your children. While I love to get outside and walk, I don't always feel like doing sit-ups or doing my ten-minute weight lifting routine. So I think of this muscle-building part much like I think about brushing my teeth. I don't especially like the time and effort it takes to brush my teeth, but I do enjoy the feeling of clean teeth.

Same with exercise. I may not always be in the mood to do my weights, but I love the feeling of my body later on. I love the fact that I burn calories at a fast rate (and can eat more). I love the way I can move and the way my clothes fit. And, typically, once I start it's easy to continue.

**The benefits of exercise are numerous:**
- Burns calories (fat)
- Builds muscles and improves muscle tone
- Increases basal metabolic rate (so you burn more calories even when you're not exercising)
- Decreases your appetite
- Gives you energy
- Fights depression and anxiety so you feel better about yourself!
- Helps you sleep better (this effect may take a few weeks)
- Reduces your risk of diabetes, cancer, arthritis, and osteoporosis
- Results in faster weight loss and better weight maintenance

How much should you do? The recommendations from the largest, most respected sports medicine and exercise organization in the world, the American College of Sports Medicine (ACSM) (www.acsm.org) suggests three different types of exercise:
- Aerobic: 20-60 minutes (in 10+ minute bouts), 3-6 days per week to burn calories, shape our bodies, and conditions the heart and lungs.
- Weight-training: 2-3 days per week to enhance strength, muscular endurance, and muscle mass.
- Flexibility training: 2-3 days per week to maintain healthy range of motion, prevent injury, and reduce muscle soreness.

Don't feel guilty if you're not doing all of that. Think of these guidelines as your long term goal. What is realistic for you to do right now? Research demonstrates that a little bit of exercise on a regular basis is better than none. A recent study reported by the New England Journal of Medicine stated that the greatest improvement in risk factors (high blood pressure, high serum cholesterol, and blood glucose levels) result from increasing the daily exercise from zero to ten minutes.

Remember that consistency is important. Don't try to cram your weekly requirement into one or two days. "Weekend warriors," who exercise long and hard on the weekend and are inactive during the week, don't do enough to build strength and are more likely to hurt their body than someone who walks 10-15 minutes a day.

Ellen used to say that she didn't have time to work out. That's because she thought that if she didn't have time to drive to the gym, workout, shower, and drive home, then she couldn't exercise. I encouraged her to change her definition of exercise away from her all-or-nothing mentality. Ellen was able to fit in a 15 minute walk every day before her morning shower.

Although many think of aerobic exercise as the most important component of exercise because it burns calories, weight-training is just as important because it builds muscles. And muscles burn more calories than fat tissue. But don't get discouraged thinking that you'll have to go to the gym to use the weights.

I've found that the easiest way to do weight-training is with exercise resistance tubes. If you've never seen them, imagine a four foot long, thick rubber band with handles on both ends. For about $10 (available at sporting goods stores), they are the most inexpensive and versatile piece of exercise equipment. As a frequent traveler, I'm not always able to make it to the gym, so I developed a workout that can be done in a six-by-six foot space. By coupling aerobic movements with eight simple weight resistance exercises and stretches afterwards, you can get a complete body workout in as little as thirty minutes. You'll find it in *Dr Jo's How to Stay Healthy & Fit on the Road* book.

Even if you don't exercise aerobically, think about making your life more active. You may want to take up gardening. It burns more calories than television, gives you something you can be proud of, and you can't eat while you are playing in the dirt. Do you have too much housework to do? Then turn up the music and dance while you clean! Here are some ideas that have worked for other people:

**How to fit exercise into your busy schedule:**
- Make it a priority by scheduling it into your day.
- Work out first thing in the morning. When you emerge from the shower, the exercise will seem just like a dream.
- Instead of sitting down to meetings, have *walking* meetings with people at work or with your family.
- Activate your daily routine. Do everything faster. Stand instead of sitting. Sit instead of lying down. Pace while you're thinking.
- Don't think "all or none." A 10-minute walk several times a day is just as good as one 30-minute walk. Walk 10 minutes in the morning, 10 minutes after lunch, and 10 minutes in the evening.
- Get on the mini trampoline while dinner is cooking.
- Exercise while you are doing something else. Do lunges while you brush your teeth. Do some stretches or sit-ups during the TV commercial. Get on the stair stepper while you watch your favorite soap operas or the nightly news.
- Reward yourself when you exercise. Treat yourself to your favorite book that you allow yourself to read *only* when you are on the stationary bike. You might forget how long you've been going!
- Listen to educational books on tape while walking or riding the stationary bike. Learn while you get lean!

- Make it fun! Take a walk in different neighborhoods and check out the landscaping. Go biking or rollarblading with your kids. Join a walking club, biking club or a competitive sports team.

Dora, the 62-year-old Mexican American woman with 13 children that I mentioned in skill #1, was not willing to change what she ate with her family. Instead, she decided to turn off the television and turn on the radio every evening and dance. Every evening her older children and their children would visit from down the street and look forward to her dances. Seven years after she lost the weight, she told me it was still a nightly routine, sometimes 2½ hours at a time.

Amy joined a health club because she thought it would motivate and inspire her to work out  - and it did. The problem was that with her family and work responsibilities she often found it difficult to get to the health club in the first place. Instead, she found a group of friends to walk in the neighborhood after the kids were in bed. This arrangement not only fit into her schedule better but offered support and motivation from her friends.

√ **Activity:**
*1. How do you plan on being more active:* _____
_____
_____

◆ **Eat adequate protein to build muscles**
Protein is important to replace the normal, daily loss of proteins from vital organs and muscle tissues - as well as to build new muscles. Most of us get the necessary amount (44 grams for women, 56 grams for men) and much more.

But I've also met clients who have cut way back on their protein because they think proteins are high in fat and calories. And they end up suffering from low energy and weak muscles. Protein, like dietary fat, helps with our satiety, the feeling of fullness. Although some dietary proteins *are* high in fat, there are many no-fat and lowfat choices that are just as high (or higher) in protein.

Each of the following "servings" contains 7-8 grams of protein:
- 1 oz poultry, fish, lean pork, lean beef, cheese *(1 oz is about the size of a chicken nugget)*
- 1 egg or ¼ c egg substitute; ¼ c fat-free or low-fat cottage cheese
- 8 oz cup of milk or yogurt
- ½ c of dried beans or peas

So you can meet your daily requirement for protein by consuming 6oz of meat (3 oz is the size of a deck of cards) and a couple glasses of skim milk or yogurt each day.

Do you "pump iron" or do aerobic workouts on a regular basis? Are you seeing better muscle tone or at least feeling stronger? If not, you may be suffering from lack of protein intake or a timing issue.

To build additional muscle mass, two things must happen. You must strengthen the muscles through exercise and you must have amino acids (the building blocks of protein) available. After you eat protein, if the body doesn't immediately need the protein, the building blocks float around for quite a few hours, but not forever. To be guaranteed that the protein you eat is available when you exercise, be sure to eat half your protein in the evening if you are working out in the morning or afternoon. Eat some protein in the morning or at lunch if you are working out before dinner. If you are working out after dinner, eat protein at both lunch and dinner. Let me illustrate why timing of protein intake is so important.

Sheila, a 21-year-old client, was at her ideal weight but was concerned about the "excessive cellulite" on the back of her legs. I thought it was unusual. Not only was she young and at her ideal weight, she had been doing a one-hour aerobic class five times a week right after work for many years.

She ate very little for breakfast and lunch (under 500 calories total). Breakfast was a banana and a slice of toast while lunch consisted of just an apple and a salad with low-fat dressing. Very little protein was consumed in the day. She had her biggest meal after working out.

I was concerned that while her daily protein intake was adequate, almost all of it was consumed *after* the workout. There may not have been enough protein circulating in her body for a workout nearly 22 hours after her high protein meal! She started eating more protein during the day and it made a significant difference in her leg's muscle tone - and she felt stronger.

If your protein intake is adequate, but you're still not seeing any results with exercise there may be other reasons. If you're very heavy, it just may be difficult to see it under the fat layer. Do you feel any stronger? If so, you're probably on the right track. If you're at a normal weight, consider the fact that you may not be feeding yourself *enough*. Just as important as protein intake, you need to make sure you're eating enough calories. Think of calories as the fuel that's needed to make the muscles in the first place. Try working on getting more calories in *before* the workout rather than *after*.

The more muscle mass we have, the leaner we look and the stronger we feel. Since muscles weigh more than fat, the scale may not immediately change once initiating exercise. An increased muscle mass will help raise our metabolism. And the higher our metabolism, the faster we lose can weight. Or if we are at our ideal weight, a higher metabolism allows us to eat more calories!

# Dr. Jo's No Big Deal Diet

## √ Activity:

*2. How much protein are you eating in a typical day?*

| Protein Foods | Servings Per Day |
|---|---|
| 1oz poultry, fish, pork, or beef (3 oz is about the size of a deck of cards) | _____ |
| 1 egg or ¼c egg substitute | _____ |
| 1oz cheese (1 sandwich slice or 1" cube) | _____ |
| ¼c cottage cheese | _____ |
| 1c (8oz) milk or yogurt | _____ |
| ½c beans or peas (ie. pinto, red, split, broad, black beans – not green beans or green peas) | _____ |

*3. Are you getting 6-8 servings of high-quality protein each day?*_____

*4. At what meals/snacks are you eating most of your protein intake?* _____
_____

*5. When do you typically workout?* _____

*6. Do you need to change when you eat your protein or when you workout?* _____
_____
_____

*7. Where can you increase or decrease your protein intake?* _____
_____
_____
_____

## Jumpstart Your Day

If you're already eating breakfast, keep up the healthy habit. Many research studies have shown that breakfast-eaters tend to be leaner than breakfast-skippers. Why? Because our metabolism slows down the longer we go without food. When we break the fast with breakfast, it jump-starts our metabolism. Eating breakfast will actually allow you to eat *more* calories!

If you're not eating breakfast, why not? Not hungry? That's probably because you're eating well into the evening and your stomach is still full. But does it make sense to eat most of your calories in the evenings when you are the least active and, thus, burning the fewest calories? Absolutely not.

Do you skip breakfast so you can enjoy the calories later on? Sounds like a valid approach, but it doesn't work that way. Breakfast jumpstarts your metabolism so if you skip it, you won't burn as many calories. Bummer! Secondly, have you ever gotten the I-need-a-siesta feeling mid-afternoon? Chances are, after skipping breakfast, you found yourself overly hungry – and overdid the lunch. A large lunch can cause a drop in your blood sugar leading to a mid-afternoon energy slump.

Some people have noted that when they eat breakfast, their stomach begins to growl around midmorning. You too? Remind yourself that it's a sign that your metabolism is picking up. Yippee! Play around with breakfast to find foods that *hold* you longer. If the cereal doesn't stick with you, try cheese toast – just broil some low-fat cheese on a slice of toast. While there are few healthy fast food breakfasts, McDonald's® Egg McMuffin® is about 300 calories and has just 12 grams of fat.

**Space Out Your Calories!**

Our bodies burn calories 24 hours a day, but we burn more during the day when we are the most active. Yet, so many people eat the majority of their calories in the evening hours rather than throughout the entire day. How do you space out your calories?

It's important to space your calories throughout most of your waking hours for a couple of reasons. First, when you eat very little for breakfast and lunch, it's only natural that you feel overly hungry in the evening. When SueAnn came to see me, she thought she had a psychological problem. She wasn't hungry for breakfast so she skipped it. Then, she often got too busy at work to eat much of lunch. On the way home from work, SueAnn would workout at the gym. But, upon returning home, she told me that her hunger and eating was totally out of control. She often didn't take the time to prepare a healthy dinner, since she was too hungry. SueAnn said that she would just stand in the pantry and eat anything on the shelves.

SueAnn's problem, though, wasn't psychological. She was simply *physically* hungry. While we burn calories all day long, we burn more calories while we are awake and active. Sure, she wasn't hungry in the morning - she had binged the evening before. And, like many of us, SueAnn had learned how to ignore her hunger as it was building up throughout the day. We tell ourselves we are too busy to eat. Or perhaps we (inaccurately) think that if we start eating early in the day, we'll only eat more as the day goes on. But that's not true. Once we get into the pattern of eating three meals a day (and healthy snacking if you'd like), your body will begin to feel satisfied and not set you up for losing control.

But there's also another reason to space your calories throughout the day. Your body burns calories 24 hours a day and needs to be fueled on a regular basis. For a simple illustration, let's say you need 2400 calories to maintain your current weight. Although our calorie expenditure is greatest when we are the most active, for this example let's just estimate that (since there are 24 hours in a day) you are burning roughly 100 calories an hour.

So what happens when you eat a 1000-calorie meal (medium-sized burger, fries, and soda) in one sitting? Since it takes just five hours to fully digest and utilize the meal, only about 500 of those calories will be burned for energy (based on our estimate of about 100 calories per hour). What happens to the other 500 calories? Well, they don't just float around the blood waiting until they're needed! Nor do they go to your muscles. Since we don't store a significant number of calories in any other form in our body, the other 500 calories have no choice but to be changed into fat.

How many times have you asked your body, when you skip breakfast, to ignore the hunger and just burn off your excess fat? Does it work? No! That's why you don't want to eat more than your body can effectively utilize at a given time.

Think about spreading your calories throughout the day. A good guideline is to eat at least half of your calories *before* you get home from an eight-hour work day. For example, if you plan on eating about 1600 calories a day, make sure you get at least 800 calories during your first 8 waking hours. If you don't, you may overeat in the evening hours, just before you go to bed! Since that's when we need the fewest calories, it's likely to keep your weight up.

That still leaves you half your calories to enjoy in the evening hours. Chances are, if you've read enough diet books, you've read that it's bad to eat after dinner. And that's fine if that rule works for you.

I decided in my eating disorder recovery, that it didn't work for me. Personally, I *always* have a nighttime snack. It prevents me from the last-supper-syndrome. Remember, that's when you think of a meal as your very last for a long time. It's much like when you pig-out before you start yet another "diet." Have you ever done that?

## √ Activity:
Think about your typical eating pattern and answer these questions:

*8. How are your calories spaced out now?*_____
_____
_____

*9. Are you eating at least half your calories by the time you arrive home after work?*_____
_____

*10. What changes could you make to spread your calories more equally throughout the day?* _____
_____
_____

# Dr. Jo's No Big Deal Tips for Accelerating Your Metabolism

1. Burn more calories through movement so you can eat more. While aerobic exercise burns calories during the session and shortly after, muscle strengthening exercise builds muscles 24 hours a day!

2. Always eat breakfast to jump-start your metabolism.

3. Space your calories out throughout your waking hours so you are burning calories most efficiently.

## My Notes:

# Skill #6:
# Ask Yourself Why

One woman shared with me her "secret" for weight loss. She said it was "simple" - she just kept a daily food record of everything she ate. I, initially, assumed she using it to monitor her calories. "No," she said. "I just write down everything I eat. If it takes up too much space, I figured I'd eaten too much and I would stop."

Believe it or not, just keeping food records is enough to help many keep their food intake on a conscious level and keep it in control. Others keep a food records to calculate the calories eaten, to count the number of fruits and vegetables eaten, or to see if you're getting enough protein.

But if you want to get to the core of what's causing you to eat more than your body needs, it's helpful to figure out why you're eating what you're eating. While you won't lose weight any faster by examining why you eat, research shows you'll be more likely to keep off the weight. And keeping the weight off means never having to be on a diet again!

Eating doesn't happen all by itself. It's always preceded by something. Sometimes it is hunger. But more often it is preceded by a signal or association such as a person, place, activity, time, a sight, or smell. It may initiate from an emotion or even the way in which you talk to yourself. If you neglect to examine the underlying reasons *why* you eat more than your body needs every day, you'll relapse in stressful situations and/or when your daily patterns change.

**Discover the Reasons Why You Eat**

When I've suggested clients keep track of what they eat, most say it takes too much time. But, does it really take more than a few minutes? No! So, give it a try.

√ *Activity:*
*1. Keep a food diary for at least a week or two. Every time you eat or drink something, note the time of the day, what you ate or drank (with specifics and amounts), where you ate, and who else was with you. Then in the last column, jot down why you ate it (such as "it was there," "I was hungry/thirsty," "it was dinnertime," "it smelled good," "I was bored," " I like them"). Then using the Hunger Scale from skill #4, note your hunger level before eating. Don't worry if you don't immediately know the "why." As you keep food records, your reasons will become more obvious.*

**Food Record:**

| Time | Food/Drink Consumed | Where & with Whom? | Why? | # on Hunger Scale |
|------|---------------------|--------------------|------|-------------------|
|      |                     |                    |      |                   |

# Dr. Jo's No Big Deal Diet

## √ Activity:

*2. After keeping the food records, try to analyze what cues, other than true hunger, played a role in what you ate and drank. The following list may provide you with some hints; although there may be other cues. Check off which ones apply to you and your eating patterns.*

## Eating Cues:

| Situations | Food | Time | Emotions |
|---|---|---|---|
| ☐ At work | ☐ Being in the kitchen | ☐ Breakfast | ☐ Elated |
| ☐ With friends | ☐ Food in sight | ☐ Mid-morning | ☐ Happily content |
| ☐ Specific people | ☐ While cooking | ☐ Lunch | ☐ Excitement |
| ☐ TV | ☐ While cleaning dishes | ☐ Mid-afternoon | ☐ Sad |
| ☐ Reading | | ☐ After work | ☐ Dis-appointed |
| ☐ Shopping | ☐ Finishing others' leftovers | ☐ Dinner | ☐ Depressed |
| ☐ Movies | | ☐ Evenings | ☐ Tired |
| ☐ Ball games | ☐ Certain smells | ☐ Workdays | ☐ Upset |
| ☐ Social events | ☐ In restaurants | ☐ Weekends | ☐ Angry |
| ☐ Vacations | | ☐ Middle of night | ☐ Frustrated |
| ☐ Meetings | ☐ At buffets | | ☐ Bored |
| ☐ Parties | ☐ Meals paid by others | ☐ Overeat at every meal | ☐ Frantic, overwhelmed |
| ☐ Holidays | | ☐ After I've skipped meals | ☐ Rejected |
| ☐ Family Gatherings | ☐ Specific foods: | | ☐ Helpless |
| | | | ☐ Stressed |

---

If you feel like you are eating too much because of any of these cues, you'll want to break the chain. How? You have many options that fall into two broad categories. You can either:

1. Eliminate or decrease that which prompts you to eat *or*
2. Substitute a new activity instead of eating.

For example, if having cookies in the house prompts you to eat them, there are many solutions. One may be to not buy them (eliminate the prompt). Or if you notice that stressful situations increase your cravings for cookies, learning to manage your stress will be helpful. You can also substitute activities by eating something lower in calories that would also satisfy you, or by taking a walk. By keeping your overeating triggers at a minimum, you'll learn to listen to your hunger.

## Eliminate or Decrease the Stimulus to Eat

Does just being in the kitchen prompt you to eat? Perhaps you weren't even hungry but you went into the kitchen to get someone else a drink or cook a meal. And there you see a food that is enticing - and you eat it. Gloria had that problem. She told herself that she wanted to start walking everyday after work. But each time she came in through the garage, which opened directly into the kitchen, she thought about eating instead of exercising. She told me that she went straight into the pantry and had no idea what she ate.

Gloria came up with a creative way to decrease the stimulus to eat by simply bypassing the kitchen. Instead of parking in the garage, she parked her car at the front of the house, came in the front door, and went directly to the bedroom (bypassing the kitchen) to change into her walking clothes. Believe it or not, it worked! Gloria eliminated the prompt to eat by changing her course in her house. And she found that walking helped her to decrease her stress - the reason she overate in the first place.

If you eat while you are doing other activities, you'll tend to associate the two of them together at an unconscious level. If you eat at the movies or while watching television, you'll automatically think about food when you turn on the television or go to a movie - even if you're not hungry.

**To keep the food/activity associations to a minimum:**
1. Eat in a calm environment
2. Eat only when sitting at the table (not at your desk, in the car...)
3. Reduce distractions; do not read or watch television while eating
4. Pay attention to the food while eating; eat slowly and savor each bite
5. Stop before you are "full" - aim for a five or six on the hunger scale rather than a ten

**Here are some other ideas to decrease the stimulus to eat:**
- Don't keep tempting foods in the house. If your kids want certain foods that you have a difficult time resisting, consider giving them money to buy it at school.
- Store tempting foods so that you can't see them. Let others keep their goodies in a cupboard that you don't always use.
- Change routes to avoid places that tempt you.
- Let others cook for themselves and get their own snacks.
- Avoid people who encourage you to overeat.
- Don't shop when you are hungry and always shop from a prepared list. You might consider using prepared menus to help guide you.
- Take your special foods or low calorie drink to places that you might be tempted to eat foods not on your plan.
- Avoid events where overeating is too tempting.
- Watch TV in a different chair. It sounds too easy, but sitting in a different place will help break the chain if you eat while watching TV.
- In a restaurant, ask immediately for a glass of water, or a cup of coffee or tea. Ask the waitress not to bring bread/crackers or keep it on the other side of the table.
- Learn to manage stress. Although stress comes from real situations, it is mostly our perceptions that determines our reactions.

- At home, clear the table immediately after each meal. Ask others to clear their own plate, dump the leftovers, and rinse their plate under the faucet.
- Each morning think about your upcoming day; plan a course of action for situations that may be difficult. Practice these actions in your mind using the visualization technique you learned in skill #2.
- Avoid food topics in your conversations with people and don't watch TV commercials.
- Serve the food in the kitchen so bowls of food are not on the table to tempt you to reach for seconds.
- If certain people prompt you to eat, think about spending less time with them.
- Carry a water bottle so you'll remember to drink plenty of water throughout the day.
- At parties, don't sit near the food and keep a low-calorie drink in your hand.
- Change the room arrangements so you can't eat dinner at the table and watch TV
- Put groceries away immediately after bringing them home.

## Substitute Activities for Eating

There are two types of substitute activities - one involves finding a healthier way to enjoy the food or drink. The other involves coming up with activities to do *instead* of eating.

### ♦ Find a healthier way to enjoy the food or drink

Let's just say you enjoy ice cream (like I do). As mentioned in the previous section, you can decrease the stimulus by not buying the ice cream in the first place. Then if you were in the mood for ice cream, you'd actually have to go out and buy it. Sometimes that's enough to make you think twice.

On the other hand, if ice cream is one of your true pleasers, when you're hungry, stressed, or bored will you just eat something else (a teaser) with the same number of calories or more? And then, feeling unsatisfied with the substitute, would you still go out and get the ice cream?

If you decide that not buying the ice cream wouldn't work, you can always find a healthier way to enjoy it. For example, if you sit down every night to a big bowl of ice cream, you have a few more options. You can:
• Eat it in a smaller quantity
• Eat it less often
• Find a lower calorie version of the food - one that still gives you pleasure

You could use a smaller bowl every evening or go to your favorite ice cream shop and order just a scoop (less than what you'd eat at home). Or you could choose to eat it only on Friday, Saturday, and Sunday evenings - a savings of more than half the total weekly ice cream calories. Lastly, you could substitute a lower calorie ice cream (or other food) that you still enjoy. Perhaps sugar-free chocolate pudding would satisfy your craving for chocolate ice cream or maybe you can find a low-fat ice cream. You decide. The important thing is to find something that works for you. Chances are there will not only be different rules for different people, but also different rules for different situations.

If you like to eat out, get a copy of my book, *Dining Lean*. This book is filled with ways to cut the calories of your favorite menu items at nearly every restaurant without feeling deprived.

### ◆ Discover other activities to do instead of eating
Sometimes, it's just plain healthier to find another activity to do instead of eating - especially if you're not really hungry. Peggy recognized that when she got the kids off to school, she rewarded herself for surviving the hectic early morning hours, by sitting down to a box of cookies. Instead she decided to reward herself with other "feel good" activities including as reading a novel, tak-

ing a shower or bath, or laying down for 10 minutes. She had to remind herself not to feel guilty about "wasting" time because she deserved it!

**Here are some other ideas for activities to do *instead* of eating:**

- Take a walk
- Read a good book or magazine
- Sew, crochet, knit or do other handiwork
- Keep a list of household chores to do instead
- Work on your photo album
- Take a bubble bath or paint your fingernails
- Practice relaxation and visualization
- Day dream
- Take a class on how to boost your self-esteem
- Talk to yourself. Tell yourself that you deserve to be treated well
- Watch a movie or listen to music
- Don't come home right from work if that is your bad time - take a relaxing walk in the park on the way home
- Read a book of jokes or riddles; do crossword puzzles.
- Argue with the food and tell it you don't like being controlled
- Take a nap
- Develop a new hobby or take a class
- Write letters or play cards
- Call a friend
- Work in the garden

# Dr. Jo's No Big Deal Diet

## √ Activity:

*3 . Think about your problem areas from the previous activity and brainstorm about how to prevent them from ruining your weight loss plans. Be creative.*

| Problem Area | Eliminate/Decrease Stimulus (how can you decrease the urge?) | Substitute Activities (what you will do instead of eating?) |
|---|---|---|
|  |  |  |
|  |  |  |
|  |  |  |
|  |  |  |

**Other suggestions:**
- Don't set yourself up for failure. Pick just one or two problem to work on at a time. Remember, this is not a diet but a slow progression into the life you want.
- Decide which solution you want to experiment with first. Put it into actual practice and evaluate its success. If it doesn't work, go back to the drawing board.
- Be realistic. It's not going to work every time. But stick with it if you can see some progress.
- Be patient. Self-management skills take time to learn. Like playing the piano or learning to type, when practiced long enough, it becomes easier to do.
- Use visualization to "see" yourself managing your problem areas. Like an actor rehearsing their lines in their head, this technique will help you to handle these tricky situations more appropriately the next time.

## Handle Your Emotions Appropriately

Ryan says he's an emotional eater. He eats when he's hungry, sad, bored, and angry. He says there's always a reason to eat. Are there some emotions that you strongly associate with eating? It's understandable because most of us learned, at a very young age, to celebrate with food. Not only birthdays, graduations, weddings, and anniversaries, but we also celebrate good grades, good days, and the end of the work week. There's nothing wrong with celebrations, but we need to learn to celebrate without food as well.

When you're stressed, instead of reaching for food, reach for an animal to pet, a friend to talk to or hug, a dance, or a quiet evening in front of the fireplace. I find that a slow stroll or a few laps in the pool are helpful. If you're upset, identify what you're really upset about and do something constructive. It might help to release your emotions in a kickboxing or even a yoga class.

If you can't talk it out with the person you're upset with, pull out your journal and put your emotions down on paper. Research has shown that expressing yourself on paper (even if you throw it away afterwards and do nothing further) helps to alleviate your stress level. Write about it every day until you feel like you are getting it out of your system. You'll notice that each subsequent writing reveals less and less anger. Don't stuff your emotions with food!

## √ Activity:

*4. Think of alternative things (other than eating) that you can do when you're bored, depressed, stressed, or feel like celebrating:* _____

_____

_____

_____

_____

## Deal with Your (Psychological) Hunger

Have you ever had one of those days, where everything that can go wrong, does? You find yourself reaching toward the cookies. Stop! Don't become the villain in your own personal weight-loss plan. If you're following a realistic eating plan, remind yourself that the hunger you think you are feeling may not be physical. The psychological hunger comes from certain patterns or habits including stress.

## Try some simple behavior modification techniques to get you back in control:

- Drink at least eight glasses of water a day. Sometimes thirst feels like hunger.
- Get rid of the food that is haunting you - down the disposal or in the trash can. The cost of the food is nothing compared to your goal of weight-loss.

- Practice meditation to relax or take a bath or a relaxing walk. Or play a hard game of tennis or go for a run.
- Give yourself 10 or 15 minutes the night before to go over the next day's schedule. Visualize how you will succeed in overcoming temptation. Plan what you need to take for lunch and pack it!
- Keep a food diary. It can help keep you straight if you write down everything that you eat - even the things that weren't on your plan. Don't just write "blew-it" across the page. Afterwards, you may want to count up your calories so you can plan how you are going to make up for those extra calories. You can exercise more or eat slightly less the next few days. Or perhaps just think of it as a learning experience and come up with a plan for next time.
- Wait ten minutes. If the craving still does not go away, then you may decide to eat. Next time, practice this for fifteen minutes and build up to waiting a half hour or more before eating.
- Psych yourself up by reading success stories – Weight Watchers, Shape, and Woman's World magazines have some powerful stories.
- Make a list of all the reasons why you want to lose weight. Use this as a reminder when you get weak. Have another list of why you want to stay at your current weight. Which is stronger?
- Stand in front of the mirror naked and ask yourself if you really want to blow it!
- Ask for support from a friend or spouse. Be selective though because some people will sabotage you by *always* telling you that you deserve to eat whatever you want. Stay away from those people when you feel weak.
- Give yourself a planned treat at least once a week. It may help you to resist temptation for the rest of the week. Sometimes it's easier to eat your special treat "out" so that you won't have to worry about what to do with the leftovers at home.
- Look at pictures of yourself when you were leaner.

- Tune out tempting television commercials by closing your eyes or switching channels. Or tape your favorite shows and fast-forward through the commercials.
- Give in to your cravings by eating something that satisfies the craving for fewer calories. If you crave salty chips, try air-popped popcorn with buttery spray and salt. If you crave chocolate, settle for sugar-free hot cocoa or chocolate low-fat frozen popsicles.
- Take a walk in the mall. Look at the plus size stores - are those the clothes that you want to limit yourself to for the rest of your life? Is there another store that has the type of clothing you want to be able to wear?
- Get involved in something that makes you feel good. Maybe you have too much leisure time on your hands - volunteer with a charity. Or maybe you spend too much time on everyone else's needs and not your own - join a club, a study group, or take up a new hobby. These activities can make you feel good about yourself and pick you up when you need it most.
- Close down the kitchen at a certain time and don't go in there after that time.
- Go someplace where you never think of food. In the bathroom or shower? Outside walking? Swimming?
- Cook ahead of time in quantity so you spend less time in the kitchen. Then just pop your premeasured serving in the microwave for your dinner. Or buy some frozen low calorie dinners for when you don't have time to cook.
- Avoid certain isles in the grocery store such as the bakery section. What you don't see won't tempt you!
- Start the day off right. Eat a breakfast that is on your plan. Then you will feel more positive you will make it through the rest of the day. Remind yourself to focus on one day - or one meal - at a time.
- Take at least twenty minutes to finish a meal. Since it takes awhile for your brain to get the message from your stomach that you're full, it's easy to eat beyond the comfort level when you eat fast.

- Stand up partway through your meal. My daughter, jokingly, came up with the "stand up and lose weight plan." She says all you have to do is stand up part way through your meal - and check your hunger. Surely, you've experienced the feeling, after eating a large meal, that upon standing you think "Oh, I shouldn't have eaten that much." So my daughter's right - if you stand up you'll feel fullness earlier.

## √ Activity:

*5. What things can you do to control your psychological hunger:*_____

_____

_____

_____

_____

_____

_____

_____

Skill #6, *Ask Yourself Why*, is all about taking control of your surroundings, rather than have them control you. Discover why you eat and come up with some planned alternative behaviors for when you eat too much, for the wrong reasons. Remind yourself that eating (for the wrong reasons) will only make the anxiety go away for a short period of time. Afterwards, you will feel twice as bad - you'll still feel anxious but you'll also feel guilty about overeating.

Remember you are only human. Don't put yourself down if you give in and splurge anyway. Change that *slip* into a learning opportunity. Pick yourself up, brush yourself off, and get back to your plan right away. Don't wait until tomorrow or next Monday.

# Dr. Jo's No Big Deal Tips for Asking Yourself Why

1. Keep a food diary and analyze why (other than hunger) you are consuming what you do.

2. Eliminate or decrease the stimulus to feed the psychological hunger by breaking the chain of events that lead to eating.

3. Find other substitutes for eating.

4. Recognize that some of your hunger is psychological. Practice some simple behavior modification techniques to get it under control.

5. Don't scold yourself when you stray from your plan. Instead, think of the mis-step as a learning experience for the next time.

## My Notes:

Skill #7:

# Keep Your Focus

The last essential skill to help you to lose weight and keep it off, is to maintain the focus on your goal. Chances are you've heard the oft-quoted "it takes 21 days to make a new habit." I don't believe it. When you've had certain habits for years, 21 days is not enough to break it. Keeping your focus requires getting the support you need from others, monitoring your success, and having a plan for when you fall back into some of your previous habits.

## Get the Support You Need

Successful dieters often get some help from others. They asked for help from their current friends and family *or* actively searched for sources of support that they didn't have in their circle of acquaintances earlier. Some people searched out mentors who had been through this before. It could be someone from their neighborhood or workplace, but is could also be someone they watched from afar.

129

Where can you find your role model? It doesn't have to be a celebrity like Oprah. Rene told me how she had watched an acquaintance at church lose weight over a years time. After hearing about and seeing her success, she took the same approach as her friend and lost the weight slowly by making a few *no big deal* changes.

Support means different things for different people. It may come from friends and family, books and other educational resources, inspirational stories, counseling, or support groups.

**Here are some ways to find support:**
- Ask family members to keep certain foods out of the house or eat them in another room
- Find a walking or running buddy (*thank you Fred, Allen, and Christine for getting me out of bed for our Saturday morning runs for all those years*)
- Tell your partner that it helps when they compliment you
- Join a group weight management program such as Weight Watchers (even if you don't follow their program)
- Join a weight management support group such as TOPS (Taking Off Pounds Sensibly) or Overeaters Anonymous that offers support without a required food plan
- Join a support group that helps you to focus on your needs such as a group designed for codependents
- Ask loved ones not to bug or nag you about your weight or food choices (there's a difference between support and nagging)
- Find a role model (such as a friend, a relative, a coworker, a movie star) for continuing inspiration
- Read inspirational stories in magazines or listen to motivational tapes
- Take a stress management course
- Visit with a Psychologist or Registered Dietitian for professional help
- Ask the restaurant manager how the chefs prepare the food and ask for suggestions for low-fat eating (servers are not usually as knowledgable)

- Get a physical trainer to help you exercise properly and develop a program that works for you and your lifestyle
- Ask a friend or mentor for advice on how to handle a difficult situation
- Observe how others control their weight and other aspects of their life
- Watch reruns of the Richard Simmons show for inspiration
- Take an interesting class to keep your mind off snacking in the evening
- Practice a hobby to keep your hands busy and your attention away from food
- Get an exercise video so you can exercise at home when the weather is bad
- Read a nutrition book to help you understand your body's needs
- Invest in one good piece of home exercise equipment
- Buy low calorie beverages and foods that keep you on track of your goals
- Use a food/exercise diary or log
- Pet an animal; it's proven to calm you down after a stressful day. In addition, having a dog is a good excuse to take a daily walk.

## √ Activity:

*1. List some of your ideas for getting the support you need.*

_____
_____
_____

### ◆ Your Allies

There will always be things that get you feeling down. Therefore, you'll want to obtain as much support as you can from your allies. Look for people at home, in your neighborhood, at church, and at work. Think about who can help with preparing the foods you want, motivate you to exercise, provide information to help you in your goal, congratulate you on your success, and counsel you on how to break some bad habits. If you are not getting all the support you need, ask these and other people for help.

## √ Activity:

*1. List your allies (those people that can offer you support):*

| My Allies | How Do They Help? |
|-----------|-------------------|
|           |                   |
|           |                   |
|           |                   |
|           |                   |

### ◆ The Saboteurs

Not all people are helpful. Some, either directly or indirectly, sabotage our goals. I often hear "if only s/he didn't....then I wouldn't have this problem."

While this may be true, don't spend too much time trying to convince these people to change. (You already know that most people do not change). Instead, spend your time and effort on changing your reaction to these people. That may include not spending as much time with them, asking them for support and understanding in a *constructive* fashion (nagging doesn't work), changing your attitude, or making sure you get more support from your allies above to counterbalance the sabotage.

Lauren is a very overweight, thirtyish woman. Her, very slim mother, frequently comments about her weight and makes suggestions on how to get it under control. Although Lauren's mom is probably trying to be helpful, Lauren tends to get upset but not say anything. Instead, she purposely eats more to "show her." When Lauren recognized that her passive-aggressive behavior wasn't helping her with her goal, she searched for another plan of action. Lauren took an assertiveness course and began practicing things to say to her mother.

At a recent family gathering, when she put a piece of fat-free cheese on her hamburger, her mother told her she didn't need it. But Lauren was ready for this and responded without the usual emotion: "Maybe you don't think so, but I planned for this. And I would appreciate if you kept your comments to yourself." Her new assertiveness training was not only helping her handle the situations better; she felt better about herself and did not binge afterwards. And, over time, her mother made fewer comments.

Sometimes we're not so lucky. If, after some assertive communications, the comments don't stop you'll have to chose another option. Remember the first skill - *no more excuses.* You can opt to spend less time with them. But, what if the saboteur is your spouse? Your boss? I've had patients tell me they find dealing with these people so difficult that they actually *do* avoid them. Some stop visiting family members as often, others have gotten new jobs, or even gotten a divorce.

I'm not recommending such drastic measures. But, if you can't get away from the hurtful people, you'll have to learn to ignore their comments and actions so they don't bother you. Go back to skill #2 and review the section on self-talk. Practice taking deep breaths and repeating (to yourself) lines such as "they know not what they say" or whatever makes you feel better. Trust me, with practice, this really works. It also helps to have a sense of humor.

As with every aspect of *Dr Jo's No Big Deal Diet*, it's up to you to decide which is the best way of handling your difficult situations. There is always more than one way.

For example, if you're the family cook and everyone else wants their foods fried, you have a few options. You can prepare two meals; one including the foods they like and another for yourself - but this extra effort gets old fast. If you do all the shopping and cooking you could be assertive and tell them that things will be different around here and you will cook only what *you* need. But that, too, may be too stressful for some of us to implement. Often clients decide to make slow and gradual changes in the way their family eats. That may mean changing only one thing at each meal, preparing the vegetables without fat and allowing them to add butter as desired, or just preparing leaner cuts of beef, fish, and chicken *more* than fried meats, but not everyday. You have to decide what is best for you.

## √ Activity:

*2. List your saboteurs (those that make losing weight more difficult). Write down what they do or say. Brainstorm about how you can handle the situations better.*

| My Saboteurs | What They Say/Do? | How I can Handle the Situation? |
|---|---|---|
|  |  |  |
|  |  |  |

Do you need to speak up and say something? Then speak to them directly without emotion. Try the following four part script to help you get your message across clearly without destroying the relationship.

1. **Describe the situation.** So there's no confusion about what your concerns are, start the discussion by letting them know what you're talking about.
2. **Tell the effect.** Let them know what reaction their action has on you.
3. **Tell how you feel.** Not everyone is comfortable naming their feelings, but I think the message is clearer when you do. Although these people may make you angry, for best results, don't use that word in your script. Here are some other feeling words that are more descriptive: frustrated, concerned, uncomfortable, embarrassed, confused, humiliated, offended, disappointed, or shocked.
4. **Tell them what you want.** This is the most overlooked step. Typically, we tell people what they've done wrong, but fail to tell them what you want them to do next time. And don't assume that they will know - be direct.

For example, you may want to say: "Angie, I was embarrassed yesterday when you announced to the whole board that you had bought the large chairs 'just for me.' I know I've established a comfortable working atmosphere here where we joke around with each other. But I'd appreciate if comments about my weight are not openly voiced."

Or "Bob, you know I've been working on getting some weight off by getting a bit more exercise and cutting back on my portions. And I know you meant well by giving me this box of chocolates for Valentines Day. But I can't control myself with chocolates. In the future, would you please not buy me food for celebrations?"

Here's another example: "Mom, when you ask, 'Do you really need that extra serving?' It only makes me want it more. I'm uncomfortable visiting you. Would you please refrain from making comments about my eating or my weight. I'd really appreciate it."

## √ Activity:

*3. Write your script for dealing with your saboteurs:*

_____

_____

_____

_____

_____

_____

## Monitor Yourself

People who have been successful at weight loss use some type of monitoring system to keep them on their plan. Monitoring is essential for gauging our progress, determining the effectiveness of our program, and to provide motivation. Weighing is the monitoring system we often think of, but may not be the best.

For example, the scale can't determine the difference between fat and muscle. Muscle is heavier than fat, but is more compact and trimmer looking. If you've never exercised and you start, you may actually gain weight, yet notice your clothes getting looser. Here are some other things to consider when using the scale to monitor your progress.

**The Scale:**

| Advantage | Disadvantages |
|---|---|
| • Frequent weighings can help us realize that our body weight fluctuates from day-to-day even if we eat and exercise exactly the same. Our body is 60% water so a 150 pound person has 90 pounds of water! Many variables affect our present body weight. Diarrhea and diuretics such as caffeine and other medications can make us lose excess water temporarily. Salty foods, hormonal cycles, and missed bowel movements can cause a temporary increase in body weight due to the fluid changes. | • You need to get rid of 3500 calories to lose a pound of body fat. Combine that scientific reality with the fact that our body weight fluctuates from day to day, and you realize why our weight changes only slowly.<br><br>• Many home scales are not very accurate<br><br>• Some people get too hung up on the weight and feel despair with little or no change. This could set them up for a binge or to go back to their old ways. |
| • Clothing sizes are based upon at least 10 pounds per size. Using clothing size alone as a check can be disastrous to some people. They may gain 10 pounds before they notice the change in the fit of their clothing. And a gain of 10 pounds may be too stressful and cause them to "give up". | • Since our body weight fluctuates, sometimes we stray considerably from our "program" and yet show a weight loss on the scale (caused by fluid changes). This can result in undeserved euphoria. It also reinforces the idea that you can get away with eating too much. Then, of course, it catches up with us. |

**How often to weigh if you decide to use the scale?**
Unfortunately, there is no correct answer. It's whatever works best for you. Consider these:
• If weighings get you depressed, feel free to not weigh at all. Use another form of monitoring.
• If you desire, weigh as much as once a week or as infrequently as once a month since weight changes slowly.
• If you understand and accept daily weight fluctuations, you may want to weigh everyday to see the general trend. Don't get caught up in day-to-day weights. If in general, the weight is coming down, then you are making progress.

**Other possible monitors to evaluate progress:**
The weight on the scale is not the only way to evaluating your progress. Do what works best for you and your emotional makeup. Here are some other options:

• Body Fat Percentage. There are several ways to estimate your body fat percentage including the simple skin fold caliper test and underwater weighing. From knowing the body fat percentage, a professional can quickly assess your ideal body weight based on your present muscle mass. This test, done every three to six months can accurately assess changes in muscle and fat. Ask your local dietitian or health club which tests they perform.
• Body measurements. Since muscle weighs more than fat, yet is more compact, you may notice your body measurements decrease faster than your weight when you take up an exercise program.
• Clothing fit. Pick a couple of pieces of clothing and assess how they fit when you put them on and as you move in them. Good areas of judgment include buttoning your jeans, changes in which hole your belt fits in, across the shoulders as you stretch forward, and in the crotch when you bend over.
• Look at yourself naked. Notice the change in the texture and the way it moves when you do.

• Keeping objective records. As mentioned earlier, you can simply keep track of what you ate, how much you exercised, and why you ate what you did. Feel free to customize any of the forms in this book for your specific objectives and needs. Being conscious of calories is helpful, but you don't have to necessarily count calories. Some pople are successful by simply recording what they eat. Others keep an exercise log to keep them motivated and on target. If you're trying to change a specific behavior such as leaving one bite of food on the plate, you could give yourself a star or sticker for everytime you are successful. Food records are especially important if the weight starts coming back on; use them to analyze what needs to be changed.

## √ Activity:
*4. How will you monitor your progress?*_____

_____

## Keep the Lapse from Turning into a Relapse

You've put a great deal of thought into your personal weight loss program. Keep in mind that no matter how perfect your plans appear to be, you probably won't do everything exactly as you expected. Remind yourself that being a perfectionist is both unrealistic and unhealthy for long-term weight-loss success. It is both healthy and normal that you would, occasionally, stray from your usual plan of action. It's OK to have something special to eat on certain occasions or to skip a day of exercise. In fact, these should really be specified on your action plan. For example, it may be more realistic to plan to walk five days a week rather than everyday. You might opt to have your special dessert every weekend rather than just once a month.

### Distinguishing Between a Lapse and a Relapse:
Lapse: a temporary and minor slip
Relapse: to fall back or to revert to a previous state

Unfortunately, after a "bad day," many dieters label themselves as a failure and go *off* their eating program. They *perceive* just a few cookies not as a lapse, but as a relapse. This is one of the reasons success should not be judged solely on weight lost, but on other factors such as the successful handling of a difficult situation in which they often fail. If you *always* eat the whole box once you get started, and this time you eat *only* half - that's progress!

I always say, "It's not what you eat, but what you think about what you eat that makes the difference." Work on your attitudes including the what-the-heck attitude ("I've already blown it - might as well eat the rest") by using positive self-talk as discussed in skill #2. And think about your goals; perfectionistic goals will set you up for failure.

### ♦ Immediate Plan for Relapse

What do you do when you go off your plan, eat more than you had planned, and feel totally out of control? Here are six steps to keep in mind:

1.  **Dispose of the food.** Destroy the food that is taunting you by throwing it in the trash, running water over it, or putting it in the disposal. In a restaurant, ask the server to take the food away. If no one's around, pour salt heavily over the food to stop the temptation or place your napkin on top of the food. If you're mind starts to convince you that you just *can't* throw the food away, remember: "It's waste or waist - take your pick!"

2.  **Remove yourself from the situation.** If you're at a party, get yourself away from the situation and into a safe place such as another room or outside where there's no food. At home, you may decide to get into the shower (have you ever overeaten in the shower?) Or take a walk.

3. **Talk to yourself in a positive manner.** Here are some ideas: "It's over and done, now let's get back to the plan," "I didn't eat as much as I would have eaten in the past," "There's nothing I can do about it now, but a walk this evening will help." If you can't think of anything positive to say, try something generic such as "I'm getting better and better every day." Or think of something comforting that your favorite aunt or a good friend would say to you.

4. **Provide yourself with activities to do for the next hour or two.** How can you get your mind off food and your lapse? Perhaps you can get with friends, go shopping, practice a hobby, or read a novel. I used to drink a cup of hot tea as a signal that my eating was over. With some practice, it became a very calming thing to do for me. Experiment to find out what activities work best for you.

5. **Calculate the *real* situation.** Most of the time, people exaggerate about what just happened. Even eating a whole box of cookies will not put on *ten* pounds! (It's probably even less than a pound). Acknowledging what the damage really is, makes it seem less severe and is less likely to send you into a downward spiral.

6. **Evaluate how to handle the situation differently the next time.** Perhaps you'll decide not to buy the cookies. You could allow yourself one cookie everyday instead of saying that you will never eat another cookie. Or perhaps you'll only buy one-serving size packages rather than the large box so there's less to haunt you.

If you follow these six steps on a regular basis, you'll catch yourself earlier in the lapse each and every time. If you can't remember everything, don't worry. The important thing is to catch yourself when you begin to slip and do something positive to stop the downward spiral.

## √ Activity:

*5. Develop your immediate plan for a relapse:*

| Guidelines for Overeating Episodes | My Specific Plan for Overeating |
|---|---|
| 1. Dispose of the food. | |
| 2. Remove yourself from the situation. | |
| 3. Talk to yourself in a positive manner. | |
| 4. Provide yourself with activities to do for the next hour or two. | |
| 5. Calculate the real situation. | |
| 6. Figure out what to do differently next time. | |

## ♦ Long Term Plan

How many pounds will you allow yourself to gain before you do something about it? How many binges? Patrick said that he can handle one or two days of lapsing but on the third day, he calls his counselor. Sometimes he takes the day off from work to address his emotional needs.

Some people say they don't worry until they're up ten pounds. Others know when a particular item of clothing gets too tight, they need to get back to asking themselves the questions in this workbook. Be honest with yourself. How much room can you give yourself before you need to get serious again?

## √ Activity:

*6. Determine your long term plan:*

*How many pounds or binges will you allow yourself to gain before you do something about it? (See a dietitian/counselor, go back to this workbook, return to a set plan of eating and exercise)*

_____

_____

*Where will you get help?*_____

## Reward Yourself

Loving yourself, as we discussed in skill #2 *Treat Yourself Right*, also includes rewarding yourself in a healthy fashion. Unfortunately, many of us have been taught to reward ourselves (when we are tired, angry, bored, or feeling stressed out) with food or a lazy activity (skipping a workout and watching television on the couch). When used frequently, these are not rewards but self-defeating actions. Let's start thinking of healthier rewards. Find things that support your own happiness such as spending time on your hobbies and your dreams.

Did you just say to yourself that you don't have time to treat yourself to these kinds of reward? What else are you doing? Some people keep driving themselves all day taking care of everybody and everything - to avoid thinking about their own concerns. Is that you? Do you keep yourself busy just so you don't have to feel any negative feelings about yourself? Is it working? Probably not, because when things stop you'll still feel disgusted with yourself.

Lisa told me that she treats herself to a monthly massage. Sylvia leaves work at 5:30 every evening, no matter what is going on and stops by the gym to workout. Janet signed up for a ceramics class - something she always wanted to learn. David told me that he has been gaining weight steadily for years. When he got up to 230 pounds he told himself that he would not buy himself a new suit. He continued to squeeze into the suits but they made him feel uncomfortable. I encouraged him to buy one suit that he felt good in to help him keep his self-esteem up. I told him that he can always take it to the tailor after he loses the weight - and he did!

It's important to remember that we are all lean and fun-loving inside. So dedicate some time each day to your lean, fun-loving person - without feeling guilty. When you take care of that lean person inside of you, it will help you take care of the outside.

Consequences for resisting these urges or losing 5-10 pounds should be a reward but not food. Here are some ideas:
• A new outfit
• Time alone
• Put money into a jar for each goal achieved to be spent on a vacation trip
• An exercise video
• A massage
• Manicure or pedicure
• A movie
• A new book

### √ Activity:
7. *My rewards for keeping to my action plan include:*_____
_____
_____
_____

Skill #7 focused on asking for help from our allies and learning how to deal with the sabateurs. You've identified a way to monitor your progress and a plan for when you lapse away from your plan. And, lastly, you've come up with rewards other than food.

# Dr. Jo's No Big Deal Tips for Keeping Your Focus

1. Don't be afraid to ask for help. Reach out to your allies.

2. Learn how to deal with the saboteurs in your life - avoid them, don't let them bother you, or say something to them.

3. Choose a way to monitor yourself - on the scale, with your clothing, using objective measures like a food diary, or another.

4. Have a plan for the lapses so they don't turn into a relapse.

5. Reward your hard work with something other than food.

## My Notes:

# Summary

Congratulations! You're on your way to a normal, healthy weight – for the rest of your life. But remember, you need more than willpower to reach your goals, you need a plan that incorporates the seven skills for successful weight loss.

Take the time, right now, to take your notes in this book and write them down on these next few pages. Don't feel like you have to work on every single one of these things at the same time - do the things that are *No Big Deal*. Then keep your action plan with you at all times to remind you of your goals. I have faith in you!

## My Action Plan for Successful Weight Loss

### Introduction:

1.   Is this the right time for me to lose weight?   •Yes  • No
If no, why not?_____
What do I need to work on before continuing?_____

_____

### Skill #1 - No More Excuses:

2.   What excuses have I been using in the past? Are they real or is there something I can do? _____

_____

What are some of the "No Big deal" changes I can make?
_____

### Skill #2 - Treat Yourself Right:

3.   Do I have any negative beliefs that are holding me back from being successful?_____

_____

_____

4.   Do I ever call myself names, scold myself, blow things out of proportion, or talk about trying to lose weight? What do I say?_____

_____

5. This is the positive self-talk that I will say instead:_____

_____

_____

6. My positive affirmation that I will practice is: _____

_____

7. These situations are difficult for me:_____

_____

   When practicing visualization I will see myself saying or doing: _____

_____

8. The thin person inside wants to eat:_____
   The thin person inside me wants to do: _____
   The thin person inside me wants me to be: _____

9. I want to treat myself as if I matter. So, I will spend more time
   on these activities just for me:_____

## Skill #3 - Make Your Own Rules:

   10. When I took a look at the diets and programs that I've been
   on, I found out that these things don't work for me:_____

_____

   This is what *does* work for me:_____

_____

_____

11. When I did an in-depth analysis of some of the difficult situations, I found these possible solutions: _____

_____

_____

12. My ideal weight is: _____

13. My goal is to lose weight at a rate of ____ pounds/week. To
   achieve that I will keep my calories under _____ calories/day.

14. I have some non-weight related goals. These include:

_____

_____

_____

**Skill #4 - No More Deprivation:**

15. I will make sure that I eat fewer calories than I burn by_____

_____

(they may include: keep food records, count calories/day or / meal, follow a meal plan, ask myself if it's worth $x$ calories, exercise more, follow a few simple rules...)

16. If I choose to cut my fat grams, I'll want to keep my intake under _____gms/day.

17. Some of the "No Big Deal" changes I want to make include:___

_____

_____

18. On the hunger scale, I'll try to start eating at a ____ and stop eating at a ____.

19. Do I drink enough water or other non-caloric, non-caffeinated beverages?_____

20. I plan on increasing my fluid intake by:_____

_____

21. I will ignore my Teasers and eat my Pleasers.
   My Teasers includes:_____

_____

   My Pleasers includes:_____

_____

22. I'm not sure if these are Teasers or Pleasers, so I will sit down and really taste the following foods:_____

_____

**Skill #5 - Accelerate Your Metabolism:**

23. What I will do to be more active: _____

_____

24. Am I eating the right amount of protein at the right time of
the day? _____
This is how I plan on correcting this:_____

_____

25. Are my calories spaced out (eating breakfast and consuming
half my calories before dinner?) _____
What changes do I need to make: _____

_____

**Skill #6 - Ask Yourself Why:**

26. What prompts me to eat & what will I do about it (including
decreasing the stimulus to eat or substitute activities for
eating?_____

_____

_____

27. When I'm feeling hungry, but know it's not physical, I will
focus on doing these things: _____

_____

_____

**Skill #7 - Keep Your Focus:**

28. These are my allies and here's how they help me: _____

_____

29. These are my saboteurs and here's what they say/do. And this
is how I'll handle it better: _____

_____

_____

30. I've developed an assertiveness script for dealing with one of my saboteurs: _____

_____

_____

_____

_____

_____

31. I plan on monitoring my progress by:_____

32. If I ever feel out of control with a lapse, I will follow the six step plan below: _____

_____

_____

_____

_____

_____

33. I will reward my success with:_____

_____

_____

_____

34. Here are some additional "No Big Deal" changes I plan on making: _____

_____

_____

_____

_____

_____

_____

_____

_____

_____